Dieter Wessinghage

Pocket Atlas of Rheumatology

Translated by Gottfried Stiasny

281 Mostly Colored Figures, 9 Color Plates

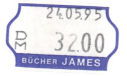

D1668567

1985
Georg Thieme Verlag Stuttgart · New York
Thieme Inc. New York

Prof. Dr. D. WESSINGHAGE, Chefarzt der Orthopädischen Klinik des BRK-Rheumazentrums Bad Abbach, Am Markt 2, D-8403 Bad Abbach/Regensburg, West Germany

Dr. G. STIASNY, Van Neijenrodeweg 574, NL-1082 HT Amsterdam, Netherlands

Library of Congress Cataloging-in-Publication Data

Wessinghage, Dieter.
  Pocket atlas of rheumatology.

  Translation of: Taschenatlas der Rheumatologie.
  Bibliography: p.
  Includes index.
  1. Rheumatism--Atlases. I. Title. [DNLM: 1. Rheuma-
tology--atlases. WE 17 W515t]
RC927.W4713 1985   616.7'23'00222   85-20853

Important Note: Medicine is an ever-changing science. Research and clinical experience are continually broadening our knowledge, in particular our knowledge of proper treatment and drug therapy. Insofar as this book mentions any dosage or application, readers may rest assured that the authors, editors and publishers have made every effort to ensure that such references are strictly in accordance with the state of knowledge at the time of production of the book. Nevertheless, every user is requested to carefully examine the manufacturers' leaflets accompanying each drug to check on his own responsibility whether the dosage schedules recommended therein or the contraindications stated by the manufacturers differ from the statements made in the present book. Such examination is particularly important with drugs which are either rarely used or have been newly released on the market.

This book is an authorized translation from the 1st German edition published and copyrighted 1984 by Georg Thieme Verlag, Stuttgart, West Germany.

Title of the German edition: Taschenatlas der Rheumatologie.

© 1985 Georg Thieme Verlag, Rüdigerstrasse 14, D-7000 Stuttgart 30, FRG
Typesetting by Druckhaus Dörr, D-7140 Ludwigsburg
Printed in West Germany by K. Grammlich, D-7401 Pliezhausen

ISBN 3-13-671601-9 (Georg Thieme Verlag, Stuttgart)
ISBN 0-86577-221-5 (Thieme Inc., New York)

Preface

Rheumatology is assuming increasing importance in medical practice as well as the hospital, both regarding the number of patients and the variety of clinical pictures and affections. This pocket atlas is primarily concerned with the clinical appearance of a number of chronic inflammatory diseases of the joints and the spine, which are of frequent occurrence and therefore present important and also characteristic alterations. To discuss the entity of pathologic alterations for the sake of completeness would mean going beyond the limits of this book. The atlas is intended for all those interested in the extensive field of rheumatology, i. e., physicians in general practice and in hospitals as well as other social institutions, medical students, and physical and occupational therapists.

The atlas also offers diagnostic clues to facilitate the differentiation between inflammatory rheumatic affections and degenerative lesions or metabolic diseases which frequently give rise to confusion and even erroneous diagnoses.

The atlas is not intended to replace a standard work on rheumatology but to complete it. The pocketbook size will allow of comparing the figures with the bedside pictures.

The present book is the result of more than 20 years' extensive scientific, and also photographic, activity in the field of rheumatology. All the photographs, with a few exceptions, have been taken by the author himself.*

The following devices and film materials were used in making the photographs:

Cameras:
1. Contarex spezial, Zeiss Ikon, Stuttgart
   Objectives:
   a) Zeiss Planar 1:2; f = 50 mm
   b) Zeiss Distagon 1:4; f = 35 mm
   c) Supplementary lenses: 1 or 2 Zeiss Proxar; f = 0.2 mm

---

* A few figures were taken from the following publications:
  Wessinghage, D.: Rheuma – Welche Diagnose stellen Sie? 2nd ed. Ciba-Geigy, Wehr 1980. Wessinghage, D.: Rheumatologie – Diasammlung und Begleittext – Erkennung und Differenzierung rheumatischer Erkrankungen. Rocom, Basel 1981.

2. Rolleiflex SL 2000, Rollei Fototechnik, Braunschweig
   Objectives:
   a) Rollei Planar 1 : 1.4; f = 35 mm
   b) Rolleinar-MC 1 : 2.8; f = 35 mm
   c) Set of extension tubes

Flashlight devices:
a) Mecablitz 163
b) Mecablitz 214
Metz-Apparatewerke, Fürth

Film material:
a) Kodachrome II K 135 15 DIN (25 ASA)
b) Kodachrome 25 135–36 15 DIN (25 ASA)
Kodak Farblabor, Stuttgart

The book could not have been completed without the assistance of my collaborators. I am greatly indebted to all parties concerned, especially my secretary Mrs. Nothaas and Dr. Zacher. On the occasion of the completion of the book I also wish to express my sincere thanks to Dr. Hauff and Mr. Menge of Georg Thieme publishers.

DIETER WESSINGHAGE
Bad Abbach/Regensburg,
October 1984

Contents

Introduction

The concept "rheumatism" covers single or manifold signs and symptoms occurring in the locomotor apparatus (the trunk and the extremities). Subjectively, there exist either trivial or troublesome dysesthesias, discomfort and painful conditions. These can appear independently or may be accompanied by swelling, deformation, malposition and ankyloses in the regions involved; they can lead to changes in the shape of parts of an extremity, entire limbs, the spine or the entire body. These isolated or associated manifestations can exert their effect on one, several or many sites of the spine and the extremities, the skeletal system and the soft tissues. Occasionally they can even affect internal organs and organ systems.

What Is Rheumatism?

Rheumatism is not a definable disease. We are concerned here with subjective and objective manifestations which, individually or in combination, can impair the patient's well-being. Localized rheumatic manifestations occur mostly in one place, but can also occur bilaterally or even in a number of places. They should be separated from acute and chronic inflammatory affections of a systemic nature. These clinical pictures can be differentiated with regard to their causes, their pathogenesis, the kind and degree of manifestation, their course and their prognosis.

What Are the Effects of Rheumatism?

Subjectively, rheumatism is characterized by dysesthesias, discomfort and pain, with or without a general sense of ill health. Objectively, there exist either discrete, and only transient, or marked, manifest swellings and possibly slight or severe deformations which can alter the shape and appearance of individual segments of an extremity, of entire limbs or the whole body.

Where Does Rheumatism Occur?

Rheumatism attacks the regions of the spine and/or the extremities. Also other, even internal, organs and organ systems are not infrequently involved.

When Does Rheumatism Occur?

Inflammatory rheumatic affections, with certain differences, are found at any age; degenerative affections develop mostly with advancing years.

The patient as well as the physician frequently interprets subjective and objective manifestations as "rheumatic" complaints without a definite diagnosis being made. However, it is precisely in the presence of rheumatic signs and symptoms that a correct diagnosis is of the greatest importance. The symptoms might be only the result of harmless local alterations, or they can constitute an acute or chronic condition of systemic, at times problematic, nature that needs a specific treatment that may be fraught with risks and complications.

Certain rheumatic lesions are frequently misdiagnosed. A typical clinical example are the multiple Heberden's nodes over the distal finger joints or the so-called Heberden's osteoarthritis in these joints. These localized degenerative lesions, most of them unsightly, occasionally painful but relatively harmless, are called gouty nodes or gouty hands and not only by the lay public. They are sometimes confused with rheumatoid arthritis or other chronic inflammatory arthropathies.

As a rule, however, there exists no relationship between this disease and gouty arthritis which is a metabolic disease. The clinical aspect alone, assisted by radiologic and laboratory studies, usually suffices to exclude this disorder.

On the other hand, an erroneous diagnosis can induce the physician to institute an ineffective or even dangerous kind of therapy. To be mentioned in this connection is the long-term use of cortisone which, occasionally, is indicated in certain forms of rheumatoid arthritis but – like the basic treatment of this disease which is not always without problems – is contraindicated in gout and in osteoarthritis of the hand or other localizations.

Apart from diagnostic and differential diagnostic criteria, familiarity with the development of typical and frequent changes in rheumatic diseases is of particular importance for their differentiation.

The Development of Chronic Types of Polyarthritis

The chronic types of polyarthritis include, among other disorders, rheumatoid arthritis of the adult with a number of subtypes to be differentiated from it, juvenile rheumatoid arthritis (of children and adelescents), psoriatic arthritis (an arthritis of a characteristic kind and localization, associated with psoriasis), and ankylosing spondylitis, in which not infrequently the peripheral joints are also affected (Table 1). The pathogenesis of these chronic arthropathies is largely unknown, although in all of them a genetic disposition is highly probable (Table 2). A genetic disposition suggests itself among other circumstances by the increased familial incidence of these disorders and the presence of certain HLA constellations. For example, the HLA-B-27 antigen can be demonstrated in 95 per cent of patients suffering from ankylosing spondylitis. The genetically predisposed organism possibly comes in contact with a multifactorial noxious agent (viruses and mycoplasmas are under debate as being primary triggering factors) which initiates a complex immunologic mechanism. In seropositive rheumatoid arthritis of the adult, an autoimmune reaction occurs, as the result of which the so-called rheumatoid factors become demonstrable. These factors form complement-fixing and complement-activating immune complexes. When these immune complexes appose themselves to the cells of the vessel walls in the synovial membranes of joints, tendon sheaths or sliding planes, an inflammatory reaction ensues. A synovitis develops in a number of structures (articular synovitis, tenosynovitis, bursitis) which gives rise to steadily increasing pathologic changes of various kind (Table 3). A long period of photographic documentation of clinical, and especially operative, findings has enabled the author to compare these lesions with one another, to describe them and to relate them to other clinical, radiologic, and histologic data. The processes developing in the joints, the tendons and in some of the bursae can be regarded as largely identical. Initially, the inflammatory lesions affect only the synovial target organ. Subsequently, however, they spread to the surrounding tissues in which they occasion secondary alterations, which, in turn, cause extensive tertiary damage.

Proliferative Phase

The immunologically conditioned damage to the synovial vessels, probably in association with the inflammation it incites, leads to increased permeability of vessel walls with transudation and exudation into the preexisting tissue spaces or potential cavities of the glide tissues in the regions of the joints, tendon sheaths and bursae. The inflammation, furthermore, stimulates the secretory activity of the synoviocytes, with which their absorptive capacity cannot keep pace. The result is the development of a hydrops in joints, tendon sheaths and bursae. Fibrin in the form of flakes or even large conglomerates precipitates in these fluid accumulations. These precipitates can, under the mechanical influence of the glide tissues, also be shaped into smaller structures, such as for example rice bodies. Pathologic proliferation caused by the inflamed synovial tissue develops concomitantly. This synovitis gives rise to multiplication and enlargement of the synovial vessels, and the entire inflamed tissue assumes a markedly reddened appearance.

Lesions of Joints

In the proliferative phase, the clinical picture of the articular lesions is characterized by swelling, frequently fusiform, of the joints involved. Proliferation of the synovial tissue and effusion can be felt on palpation (Table **33**, Fig. 1).

Roentgenograms taken in the proliferative phase reveal only anomalies of the soft tissues. In the periarticular region, the soft tissues display a frequently fusiform swelling and an increase in density of the soft tissues, which also extend to the preformed fluid-filled recesses (Table **5**, Fig. 1). The contents of the joint, which are made up of inflamed synovial tissue, effusion and fibrin, cause the lines of the articulating bones to spread and thus produce an actual widening of the so-called radiologic joint space.

Proliferation of the inflamed synovial tissue (capsular pannus), effusion and precipitation of fibrin lead to overdistention of the fibrous joint capsule and, through irritation of the pain receptors, to pain in the distended capsule. The pain gives rise to functional restriction of motion and weight bearing in the joint involved which is, however, reversible (Table **4**, Fig. 1). The tendency to inflammatory proliferation causes a thin, filmy membrane to grow across the surface of the cartilage, starting from the border between bone and cartilage (the intra-articular portion of the bone being covered with periosteum and, above it, with synovial tissue). This inflammatory synovial cartilage cover constitutes the so-called cartilage pannus. The pannus contains variable, but typical, vascular markings.

Lesions of Tendons

Tenosynovitis manifests itself by a visible and palpable swelling underneath and beside the ligaments, which more or less corresponds with the course of the tendon (Table **6**, Fig. 1). This swelling can give rise to pain-induced restriction of motion, to the phenomenon of snapping finger and later on, although less frequently, to blocking, particularly of fingers in the flexed or extended position.

On gross inspection one sees a proliferation of the inflamed synovium, similar to that observed in the joints. The proliferation develops in the synovial lining of the gliding tissues of the tendons during the proliferative phase (Table **7**, Fig. 1). This massive synovitis of the gliding structures of the tendon underneath the respective ligaments corresponds to the capsular pannus in the joint, whereas the cartilaginous pannus is identical to the filmy tendinous pannus.

Lesions of the Glide Spaces Bursae

Also in the region of the glide space between the various tissue layers, which are movable against each other, there develops an inflammatory proliferation of the synovial lining. A particular location, with its corresponding mechanical disposition, leads initially to the formation of a bursa and, during the further evolution of the chronic inflammatory arthropathies, to the development of a bursitis (Tables **2, 8, 9**).

Such a bursitis is frequently encountered at the olecranon, over the extensor surfaces of the metacarpophalangeal joints, on the medial side of the metatarsophalangeal joint of the great toe in inflammatory rheumatic or degenerative hallux valgus, over the typical plantar dislocation of the metatarsal heads in the ball of the so-called rheumatoid forefoot, and over the interphalangeal joint of a hammer toe. These bursae can be painful when they develop in an exposed area.

Destructive Phase

In this phase the synovitis, also owing to its proliferative tendency, spreads to other tissues and produces destructive damage there. Besides this active destruction, the overstretching of the contiguous tissues gives rise to passive destruction.

Lesions of Joints

In the destructive phase, similar to the proliferative phase, swelling and effusion into the joint with pain-induced restriction of function are in the forefront of the clinical picture (Table **3**, Fig. 2). These manifestations are the result of the constant increase in capsular tension, the development of an effusion and the precipitation of fibrin. The increasing pressure developing in this manner leads to overstretching of the capsuloligamental apparatus, and ultimately its permanent destruction. The synovial capsule, which often is greatly thickened, is subjected to considerable pressure and can protrude through the weakened structures: it can herniate into the upper recess of the knee joint, into the popliteal space (Baker's cyst, arthrocele), or through the dorsal aponeurosis on the extensor surface of the proximal interphalangeal joints of the fingers. Such perforation of the synovial capsule is the principal cause of the buttonhole deformity of the fingers. Larger protrusions of the joint capsule, such as Baker's cyst, contain chiefly precipitated fibrin and joint fluid, less frequently inflamed synovial tissue. When its contents increase, the cyst can extend beyond the calf. When such an arthrocele ruptures, its contents descend as far as the distal part of the lower leg and the ankle joint. This gives rise not only to discomfort but frequently to massive swelling with redness of the entire posterior aspect of the lower leg and the surroundings of the ankle joint, as well as tightness of the skin, so that the condition frequently mimics a thrombophlebitis. Mechanical impairment and pain produced by the overstretched capsule lead, also in the destructive phase to functional restriction of motion and weight bearing.

With extensive destruction of cartilage, the roentgenogram reveals a concentric narrowing of the so-called joint space, associated with haziness or disappearance of the marginal lamella. Erosions are distinctly recognizable as defects of bone (Table 5, Fig. 2). Depending on the projection, these erosions, which mostly are marginal but sometimes located more deeply, are misdiagnosed for cysts. In addition, similar to the proliferative phase, a juxta-articular osteoporosis and also thinning of the cortical bone are encountered.

Articular synovitis with formation of a cartilaginous pannus destroys the cartilage, initially by impairing its nutrition and also through enzymatic damage to the uppermost cartilage layers. The increasing, primarily planar, growth of the cartilaginous pannus with development of new vessels and their characteristic formations, then causes the pannus to perforate the deep structures, at first the cartilage itself and later on the subchondral bone. The synovitis undermines the borders of the cartilage. Following removal of the cartilaginous pannus, only slight macroscopic changes in the cartilage surface are recognizable, depending on the degree of progression. When the inflammatory activity continues, one encounters not only planar destruction of cartilage and bone but, in addition, more or less deep-reaching foci of destruction in the form of smaller or larger erosions and finally, when the disease is particularly aggressive, mutilations with defects of larger segments of joints or entire joints. A marked degree of destruction is frequently present under the collateral ligaments (Table 4, Fig. 2), at the knee joint, especially in the intercondylar fossa, and under the menisci near the tibial head. On the other hand, the destructive action of the inflamed synovial tissue does not only have an impact on the articular cartilage and the bone. At the knee joint, for instance, the synovitis proliferates to the infrapatellar fat pad and the menisci, also leading to their destruction. The medullary pannus, which contributes to the development of destructive foci, expands in the subchondral spongiosa, and also in the marrow cavity. In addition, it can break from the bony region through the cartilage into the articular surface.

Lesions of Tendons

When there is involvement of tendons or tendon sheaths in the destructive phase, physical examination likewise encounters swellings with and without crepitation along the tendons, as well as pain-induced restriction of motion in dependent parts. Temporary blocking of flexed or extended fingers occurs less frequently (Table **6,** Fig. 2). In the destructive phase, tenosynovitis – owing to its invasive growth – leads to destruction of the tendon (Table **7,** Fig. 2). Increasing structural damage can eventually cause the tendon to rupture (stabilized phase) and thus lead to complete loss of function. On performing a tenosynovectomy, the ingrowth of tissue of the inflamed tendon sheath into the tendon frequently presents considerable difficulty. It can thus happen that the tendinous pannus, which often has penetrated the tendon itself diffusely and deeply, can only be shelled out insufficiently and with additional damage to the tendon tissue (Table **7,** Fig. 2). Operative removal is, however, the only possibility of arresting further destruction. Depending on the degree of destruction already obtaining, the unavoidable removal of the inflamed synovial tissue can diminish the stability of the tendon when it is exposed to strain so that, in exceptional cases, even postoperative rupture can occur. In advanced stages, a massive conglomerate of several tendons, overgrown by inflamed synovial tissue with new formation of multiple vessels, is apt to develop. Even when individual tendons have ruptured, this conglomerate and the fact that the tendon structure is interlaced with inflamed tenosynovial tissue can largely compensate for the lost function of individual tendons. Such a compensated tendon rupture can only be diagnosed at tenosynovectomy. Additional reconstructive procedures are then needed.

Lesions of Glide Spaces/Bursae

In these tissues the destructive phase is characterized by variable, but frequently massive, swelling of the bursae. When a synovitis is present in a neighboring joint, the increasing inflammatory activity of the synovial lining of the bursae can produce destruction of the intervening tissues, thus establishing a communication between the bursa and the joint. The continually formed inflammatory fluid and the precipitated fibrin can then pass freely from the joint to the bursa, and less frequently in the reverse direction. Spontaneous closure of this communication, even following regression of the inflammatory activity, is not to be expected.

Degenerative Phase

Beside the conditions already described (in the first place synovitis and the resulting destruction), one encounters in this phase degenerative lesions as sequelae.

Lesions of Joints

Insufficiency of the destroyed capsuloligamental apparatus and destruction of cartilage and bone also lead to instability of the joint and thus to incongruity of the articular surfaces. This not infrequently results in subluxation or dislocation of the joint, but also in beginning malpositions which increase when exposed to weight bearing (Table 3, Fig. 3a). Initially, it is only the pain which restricts the function of the joint. During the further evolution of the disease, weight-bearing capacity and mobility become largely limited by the, often considerable, impairment of the articular mechanics, the faulty positions, the muscular atrophy and the secondary involvement of fasciae and ligaments.

These alterations, together with the impaired nutrition of the cartilage produced by the changing synovial milieu as the result of synovitis and the limitation of motion and weight bearing, lead to secondary para- and postarthritic osteoarthritis. The osteoarthritis progresses independently from the inflammatory synovitis, the latter may also be perpetuated (Table 4, Fig. 3b). The cartilage presents an increasing yellowish discoloration with diminution of its luster, unevenness and distortion, fraying, fissuring, and on the whole extensive wear and tear. The roentgenogram reveals hypertrophic lipping as well as spurs formed by chondrophytes and osteophytes at the border between bone and cartilage (Table 4, Fig. 3b and Table 5, Fig. 3a). The previously demonstrable osteoporosis and the thinning of the cortex increase. In addition, subchondral sclerosis develops. The roentgenogram also demonstrates the deformation of joints and the partial or total incongruity of the articular surfaces.

Lesions of Tendons

The preceding proliferation and destruction of the tenosynovial and the tendinous tissues lead to the corresponding degenerative alterations. Physical examination reveals swellings along the course of the tendons (Table 6, Fig. 3), partial adhesion and overstretching of tendons, and partial loss of function of dependent parts due to pain and occasionally to blocking with snapping fingers. These are the characteristic features of the degenerative phase. At the outset, the degenerative changes – in the presence of continued proliferation – are not infrequently recognizable by the change of the typical whitish luster of the tendons to a dull appearance with a yellowish discoloration (Table 7, Fig. 3). Impaired nutrition occasioned by alterations of the synovium, synovitis and its sequelae, produce degenerative damages to the tendons themselves and their glide way. The structure of the tendon becomes overstretched and the lesions of the glide way can give rise to partial adhesions. Structure-less appendages of connective tissue and fibrin, which cannot be differentiated macroscopically, are attached to the tendons.

Lesions of Glide Spaces/Bursae

The continually decreasing inflammatory activity is the reason for the degenerative phase, and, particularly in the following burned out phase, only instances of regressive bursitis are generally encountered. They no longer exhibit an increase in inflamed synovial tissue. The bursae, as well as the thin superjacent adhering membrane, which during the evolution of the disease frequently assumes a reddish-violaceous color, appear to be overstretched but they are still filled with fluid, the amount of which fluctuates. In this stage of development the bursae show no tendency to decrease in size or to adhesion of their parietal layers.

Burned-Out Phase

After the degenerative phase has passed, the burned-out phase of the chronic inflammatory arthropathies exhibits a regression of the inflammatory activity. The symptoms are thus cleared, but healing is only relative because of the residual defects that already are manifest and no longer reversible. Episodic flares of the disease are not to be expected in the burned-out phase, whereas in the preceding phases the inflammatory activity of the disease can return at any moment. The burned-out phase is the end stage of the inflammatory disorder.

Lesions of Joints

In the joints, the inflammatory lesions, i. e., the synovitis, undergo regression. Physical examination reveals neither swelling nor an effusion (Table 3, Fig. 4). Inflammatory destruction usually shows no further progression. In contrast, postarthritic degenerative damages, like any other osteoarthritis, continue to progress (Table 4, Fig. 4). Deformations, faulty positions, contractures that are already present do not improve spontaneously. Any resulting limitation of function is, as a rule, no longer reversible without operative intervention, but it is liable to increase in the absence of functional treatment. In the burned-out phase, the roentgenogram reveals no anomalies of the soft tissues (Table 5, Fig. 4). Degenerative (osteoarthritic) lesions already in existence continue to worsen. Exposed to constant strain, the incongruity of the articular surfaces, and possible faulty positions, which can also be due to diminished stability from collapse of parts of the joint, will increase. In addition, general osteoporosis is demonstrable.

Lesions of Tendons, Glide Spaces, and Bursae

Apart from inflammatory proliferation of the glide tissue, the burned-out phase is largely identical to the degenerative phase. Massive swelling from tenosynovitis and bursitis is no longer present, nor is an inflammatory episode to be expected. Degenerative changes of tendons and bursae, however, continue progressing (Table **7**, Fig. 4). Restriction of function, which already is manifest, can likewise persist or even increase (Table **6**, Fig. 4).

Stabilized Phase

The stabilized phase, similarly to the burned-out phase, is an end stage of rheumatoid arthritis. The condition becomes stabilized at the sites where the disease manifests itself, and sometimes even systemically. The inflammation, i. e., the active disease process, clears with residual defects. There no longer occurs any inflammatory proliferation with new damage to the tissues. The function of motion also becomes stabilized. The region involved has become immobile. The regression of function and mobility leads to elimination of the functional impulse that stimulates the synovial membrane. The latter becomes fibrotic or it involutes with formation of a scar, so that synovitis can no longer occur. The disease is thus deprived of its target organ. This stage of stabilization occasionally comes about as the result of the inflammatory process with its direct and indirect sequelae, the mechanical impairment of the pattern of motion, and the additional impact on the surrounding parts, but primarily by the patient's pain-induced inactivity.

Lesions of Joints

Especially in adult rheumatoid arthritis, the degenerative phase can give rise to so-called fibrous ankylosis of the joint (Table **3**, Fig. 5a; Table **4**, Fig. 5a; Table **5**, Fig. 5a). In contrast, bony ankylosis (Table **3**, Fig. 6b; Table **4**, Fig. 5b; Table **5**, Fig. 5b) predominantly develops from the destructive phase, skipping the degenerative phase, for example, in ankylosing spondylitis with involvement of peripheral joints, in juvenile rheumatoid arthritis, and in psoriatic arthritis. Stabilization of the joint and abolition of its mobility eliminate the functional impulse that stimulates the synovial membrane. Also in the stabilized phase, the condition clears with residual defects. When the joint becomes anky-losed in the position of function, in the knee joint it is the extended position that permits nearly painless standing and walking, the patient becomes resigned to the stiffening of the joint. On the other hand, ankylosis in an awkward position can be a major handicap. Radiologically, the stabilized phase no longer shows any soft tissue changes. In so-called fibrous ankylosis, the cartilage is largely reduced or completely absent (Table **5**, Fig. 5a). Bony ankylosis presents a fibrillar structure (Table **5**, Fig. 5b). The stabilized phase is altogether characterized by general osteoporosis due to prolonged inflammatory activity of the disease, inactivity on the part of the patient, and possibly long-term cortisone treatment.

Lesions of Tendons

On transition from the degenerative phase, tenosynovitis can give rise to partial, and ultimately complete, adhesion of the tendon to its surroundings, i. e., the tendon sheath. This occurs particularly when previously, also for other reasons, free movement of dependent parts was no longer possible. The invasive growth of the tissues of the inflamed tendon sheath in the destructive phase can ultimately be the cause of complete destruction of the tendon, resulting in its rupture. The consequence is complete loss of function of the muscle with its tendon, which cannot even be compensated for by the dependent segment of the extremity (Table **6**, Fig. 5; Table **7**, Fig. 5).

Lesions of Glide Spaces/Bursae

When bursitis has been followed by adherence of the deep and the superficial leaf of the bursa, the glide space is no longer capable of functioning (Tables **8** and **9**). The developing cicatricious fibrosis permits no movement between the two adjacent layers. Clinically, the region of the past severe bursitis presents extensive, more or less indurated, rudiments that are largely fixed to the skin. Isolated pea-sized or bean-sized rounded structures, which also are indurated but can readily be delimited from the previous wall of the bursa, are rheumatoid nodules.

Color Plates

Table 1 Frequent Chronic Inflammatory Affections of the Joints and the Spine

Table 2 Developmental Mechanism of Polysynovitis; Articular Synovitis – Tenosynovitis – Bursitis

Noxious agent

Organism with genetic predisposition

Polysynovitis

Tendon sheath: **tenosynovitis**

Joint: **articular synovitis**

Bursa: **bursitis**

Table 3 Development of Articular Synovitis – Clinical Picture

Proliferative Phase
Swelling, effusion into the joint, pain-induced limitation of function (Fig. 1)

Inflammatory episode

Destructive Phase
Swelling, effusion into the joint, pain-induced limitation of function, infrequently synovial herniations (Baker's cyst etc.) (Fig. 2)

Burned out Phase
No swelling, no effusion, deformation, faulty position, contracture, major limitation of function (Fig. 4)

Degenerative Phase
Swelling, effusion into the joint, crepitation, synovial herniations, instability, faulty position, impairment of function (Figs. 3a and b)

Stabilized Phase
Fibrous or bony ankylosis, often in a non-functional position, loss of mobility (Figs. 5a and b)

Table 3 (continued)

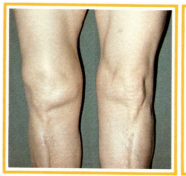

Fig. 1   Proliferative Phase
Swelling, effusion into the joint, pain-induced limitation of function

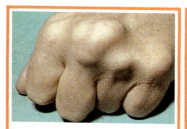

Fig. 2   Destructive Phase
Swelling, effusion into the joint, pain-induced limitation of function. Infrequent occurrence of synovial herniations (Baker's cyst etc.)

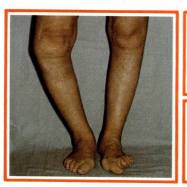

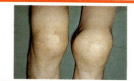

Figs. 3a and b   Degenerative Phase
Swelling, effusion into the joint, crepitation, synovial herniations, deformation, instability, faulty position, impairment of function

Table 3 (continued)

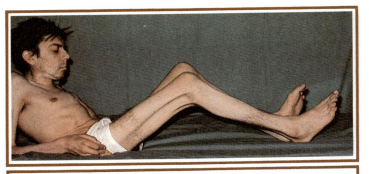

Fig. 4   Burned out Phase
No swelling, no effusion, deformation, faulty position, contracture, major limitation of function

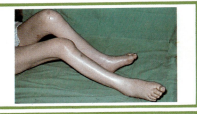

Figs. 5a and b   Stabilized Phase
Fibrous or bony stiffening (anky-losis), frequently in non-functional position, loss of mobility

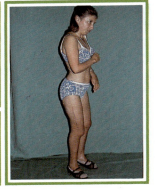

Table 4   Development of Articular Synovitis – Macroscopic Picture

Proliferative Phase
Synovitis: capsular pannus, cartilage pannus (Fig. 1)

Inflammatory episode

Destructive Phase
Destruction due to synovitis: cartilage, bone, fibrous capsule (Fig. 2)

Burned out Phase
No active synovitis, progressive postarthritic secondary osteoarthritis (Fig. 4)

Degenerative Phase
Active synovitis, para- and postarthritic secondary osteoarthritis (Figs. 3a and b)

Stabilized Phase
Stabilization of function and local stabilization of the disease process through bony ankylosis and so-called fibrous ankylosis (Figs. 5a and b)

Table 4 (continued)

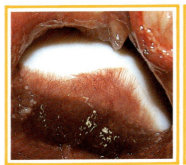

Fig. 1 Proliferative Phase
Synovitis: cartilage pannus, capsular pannus

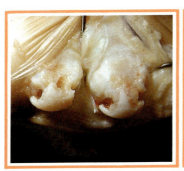

Fig. 2 Destructive Phase
Destruction due to synovitis: cartilage, bone, fibrous capsule

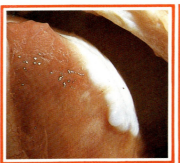 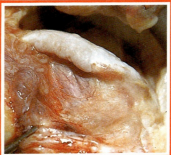

Figs. 3a and b Degenerative Phase
Active synovitis: para- and postarthritic secondary osteoarthritis

Table 4 (continued)

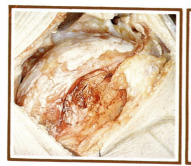

Fig. 4 Burned out Phase
No active synovitis, progressive postarthritic secondary osteoarthritis

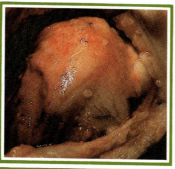 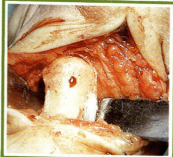

Figs. 5a and b Stabilized Phase
Stabilization of function and local stabilization of the disease process through bony ankylosis and so-called fibrous ankylosis

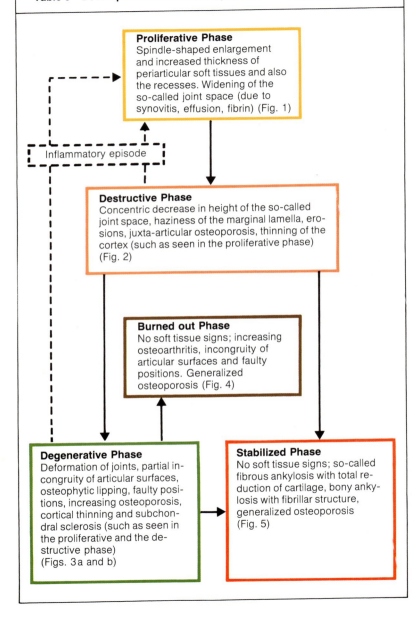

Table 5   Development of Articular Synovitis – Radiographic Picture

Proliferative Phase
Spindle-shaped enlargement and increased thickness of periarticular soft tissues and also the recesses. Widening of the so-called joint space (due to synovitis, effusion, fibrin) (Fig. 1)

Inflammatory episode

Destructive Phase
Concentric decrease in height of the so-called joint space, haziness of the marginal lamella, erosions, juxta-articular osteoporosis, thinning of the cortex (such as seen in the proliferative phase) (Fig. 2)

Burned out Phase
No soft tissue signs; increasing osteoarthritis, incongruity of articular surfaces and faulty positions. Generalized osteoporosis (Fig. 4)

Degenerative Phase
Deformation of joints, partial incongruity of articular surfaces, osteophytic lipping, faulty positions, increasing osteoporosis, cortical thinning and subchondral sclerosis (such as seen in the proliferative and the destructive phase) (Figs. 3a and b)

Stabilized Phase
No soft tissue signs; so-called fibrous ankylosis with total reduction of cartilage, bony ankylosis with fibrillar structure, generalized osteoporosis (Fig. 5)

Table 5 (continued)

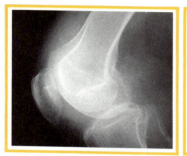

Fig. 1   Proliferative Phase
Spindle-shaped enlargement and increased thickness of periarticular soft tissues, including the recess. Widening of the so-called joint space (due to synovitis, effusion, fibrin)

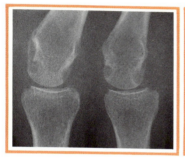

Fig. 2   Destructive Phase
Concentric decrease in height of the so-called joint space, haziness of the marginal lamella, small areas of bone erosion, juxta-articular osteoporosis, cortical thinning, subchondral sclerosis (such as seen in the proliferative phase)

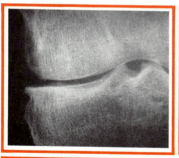
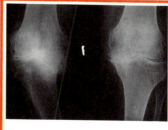

Figs. 3a and b   Degenerative Phase
Deformation of joints, partial incongruity of articular surfaces, osteophytic lipping, faulty positions, increasing osteoporosis, cortical thinning and subchondral sclerosis (such as seen in the proliferative and the destructive phase)

Table 5 (continued)

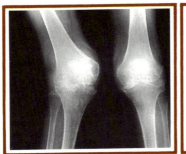

Fig. 4 Burned out Phase
No soft tissue signs. Increase in osteoarthritis, incongruity of articular surfaces and malpositions. Generalized osteoporosis

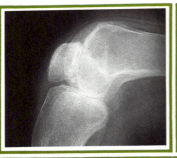

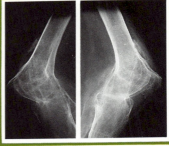

Fig. 5 Stabilized Phase
No soft tissue signs; so-called fibrous ankylosis with total reduction of cartilage, bony ankylosis with fibrillar structure, generalized osteoporosis

Table 6   Development Tenosynovitis – Clinical Picture

Proliferative Phase
Swelling along the course of the tendons, pain-induced limitation of motion (Fig. 1)

Inflammatory episode

Destructive Phase
Swelling along the course of the tendons, pain-induced limitation of motion. Temporary blocks infrequent (Fig. 2)

Burned out Phase
Limitation of motion and blocks following preceding swelling (Fig. 4)

Degenerative Phase
Swelling along the course of the tendons, pain-induced limitation of motion, blocks, adhesion and overstretching (Fig. 3)

Stabilized Phase
Complete or partial impairment of motion following rupture or total adhesion (Fig. 5)

Table 6   (continued)

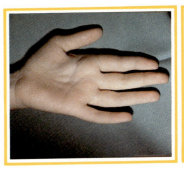

Fig. 1   Proliferative Phase
Swelling along the course of the tendons, pain-induced limitation of motion

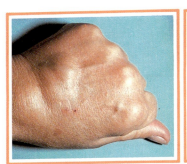

Fig. 2   Destructive Phase
Swelling along the course of the tendons, pain-induced limitation of motion. Temporary blocks infrequent

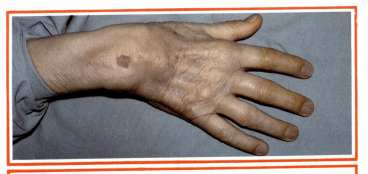

Fig. 3   Degenerative Phase
Swelling along the course of the tendons, pain-induced limitation of motion. Temporary blocks infrequent.

Table 6 (continued)

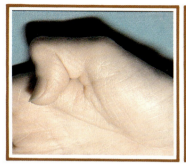

Fig. 4 Burned out Phase
Limitation of motion and blocks
following preceding swelling

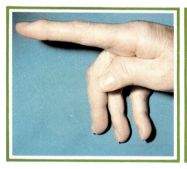

Fig. 5 Stabilized Phase
Complete or partial impairment
of motion following rupture or
total adhesion

Table 7   Development of Tenosynovitis – Macroscopic Picture

Proliferative Phase
Synovitis: tendinous pannus
(Fig. 1)

Inflammatory episode

Destructive Phase
Destruction due to synovitis:
tendons, ligaments (Fig. 2)

Burned out Phase
No active synovitis. Progressive
overstretching (Fig. 4)

Degenerative Phase
Active synovitis, overstretching
of tendons with destructive
changes, partial adhesion of
tendons (Fig. 3)

Stabilized Phase
Stabilization of function and local
stabilization of the disease process as the result of tendon rupture and total adhesion of tendons (Fig. 5)

Table 7 (continued)

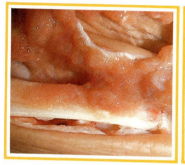

Fig. 1 Proliferative Phase
Synovitis: tendinous pannus

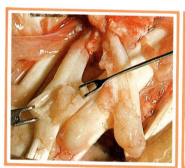

Fig. 2 Destructive Phase
Destruction due to synovitis:
tendons, ligaments

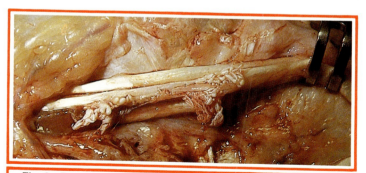

Fig. 3 Degenerative Phase
Active synovitis; overstretching of tendons with destructive
changes, partial adhesion of tendons

Table 7 (continued)

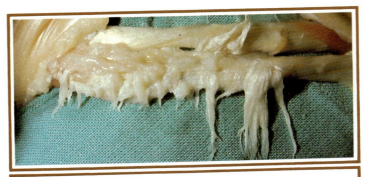

Fig. 4 Burned out Phase
No active synovitis. Progressive overstretching

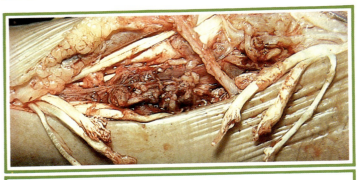

Fig. 5 Stabilized Phase
Stabilization of function and local stabilization of the disease process as the result of tendon rupture and total adhesion of tendons

Table 8   Development of Bursitis – Clinical Picture

Proliferative Phase
Massive, although not always fluctuating swelling, occasionally associated with redness and increased heat in exposed places

Inflammatory episode

Destructive Phase
Rubbery bursitis as well as synovitis of the neighboring joint, distinct fluctuation of fluid alternating between bursa and joint because of communication

Burned out Phase
Bursa with increased thickness of its wall and slight but variable accumulation of fluid; signs of inflammation absent and not to be expected in the future

Degenerative Phase
Distinctly episodic occurrence of bursitis with presence of fluid. The overlying skin is thin, shiny and livid-red

Stabilized Phase
Loss of the gliding capacity of the tissue layers separated by the bursa due to replacement of the bursa by a fibrotic scar

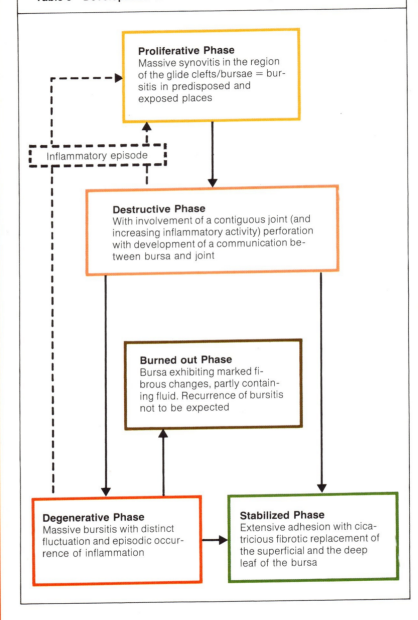

Table 9 Development of Bursitis – Macroscopic Picture

Proliferative Phase
Massive synovitis in the region of the glide clefts/bursae = bursitis in predisposed and exposed places

Inflammatory episode

Destructive Phase
With involvement of a contiguous joint (and increasing inflammatory activity) perforation with development of a communication between bursa and joint

Burned out Phase
Bursa exhibiting marked fibrous changes, partly containing fluid. Recurrence of bursitis not to be expected

Degenerative Phase
Massive bursitis with distinct fluctuation and episodic occurrence of inflammation

Stabilized Phase
Extensive adhesion with cicatricious fibrotic replacement of the superficial and the deep leaf of the bursa

Brief Survey of the History of Rheumatology

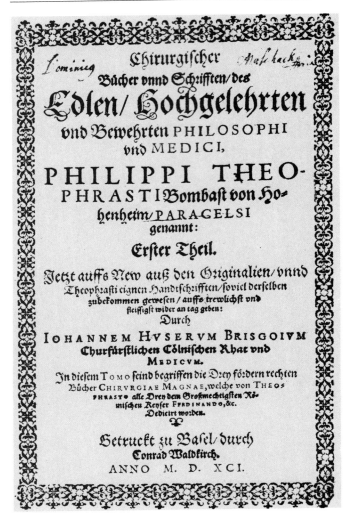

1a

Figs. **1a–c** *Theophrastus von Hohenheim,* called *Paracelsus* (1493–1541)
was one of the great reformers of medicine in that he used naturalistic thinking
in medicine and pharmacology. He distinguished between arthritic and rheumatic conditions. He regarded the passage of "tartarus" (tartaric acid) from the

Der Grossen Wundtartzney

Das Erste Buch:

Deß. Ergründten vnd Bewehrten / der
Beyden Artzney DOCTORIS
PARACELSI,

Von allen

Wunden/Stich/Schütz/Brändt/Thierbiß/
Beinbrüch/vnd alles was die Wundtartzney begreifft/
mit gantzer Heylung / vnd Erkänntnuß aller Zufäll/
gegenwertiger vnnd künfftiger / ohn allen gebresten.
angezeig: von der Alten vnd Newen Kün-
sten Erfindung /nichts vnter-
lassen:

Geschrieben

Zu dem Großmechtigsten / Durchleuchtig-
sten Fürsten vnd Herrn/Herrn Ferdinanden/ꝛc.Rö-
mischen König / Ertzhertzogen zu
Osterreich/ꝛc.

Außgetheilt in drey Tractaten.

Der Erst/in die Erkanntnuß der Wunden/was we-
sens sie gegenwertig seyend/wz zukünfftigs zuerwar-
ten/mit sampt allen Zufällen.

Der Ander/von aller Heylung/ so je vnnd je bey den ge-
rechten Artzten gebrocht / von anfang der Artzney/
biß auff die jetzig gegenwertige zeit.

Der Dritt / von dem Biß vnnd Hecken der vergifften
Thier/Beinbrüch/alle arth deß Brandts/vnnd was
dergleichen der Wundartzney zustehet/innhalt.

1 b

a ij

blood into the joints as the cause of gouty arthritis. The designation "arthritis" was first used by Galen (AD 131–201) as a comprehensive term for all inflamed joints.

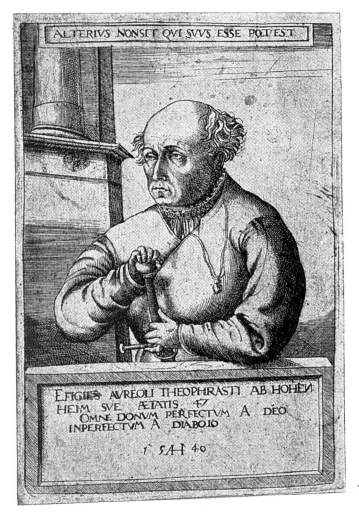

ALTERIVS NONSIT QVI SVVS ESSE POTEST

EFIGIES AVREOLI THEOPHRASTI AB HOHEN
HEIM SVE ÆTATIS 47
OMNE DONVM PERFECTVM A DEO
INPERFECTVM A DIABOLO

1 5 4 0

1c

DEMETRII

PEPAGOMENI, LI-

BER DE PODAGRA, ET ID GE-
NVS MORBIS.

Ad imperatorem, Michaëlem Palæologum.

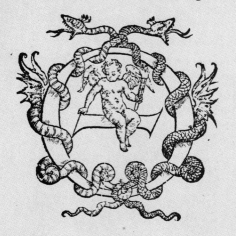

PARISIIS, M. D. LVIII.

Apud Guil. Morelium, *in* Græcis *typo-
graphum* Regium.

PRIVILEGIO REGIS.

2

Fig. **2** Treatise dedicated in 1558 to the Byzantine emperor *Michael Palaeolo-
gus,* who perhaps had gout.

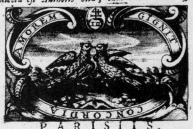

GVLIELMI

BALLONII

MEDICI PARISIENSIS CELEBERRIMI,

CONSILIORVM

MEDICINALIVM LIBRI II.

A IACOBO THEVART, Facultatis Medicæ Parif. Doctore,
Authoris pronepote, fcholiis nonnullis illuftrati,
digefti ac in lucem primùm editi.

TOMVS PRIMVS.

In quo pleraque continentur quæ & ad Morborum cognitionem,
eorumdemque curationem propofitis Exemplis, & obfcurorum
Hippocratis locorum intelligentiam pertinebunt.

Inter cetera elegantiffimum & vtiliffimum eft de Calculo Opufculum.

Adiecta eft Authoris vita, cum Indicibus neceffariis.

PARISIIS,

Apud IACOBVM QVESNEL, viâ Iacobæâ,
fub figno Columbarum.

M. DC. XXXV.
CVM PRIVILEGIO REGIS.

3a

Figs. **3a–d** The Parisian physician *Guglielmus Ballonius (Guillaume de Bail-
lou)* (1538–1616) coined the concept of rheumatism giving a detailed description of the articular symptoms in rheumatic fever and differentiating them from
those in gout. He also mentioned sciatica.

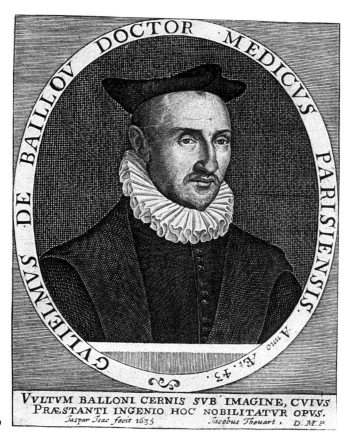

GVLIELMVS DE BAILLOV DOCTOR MEDICVS PARISIENSIS.

A^{no} Æt. 45.

VVLTVM BALLONI CERNIS SVB IMAGINE, CVIVS PRÆSTANTI INGENIO HOC NOBILITATVR OPVS.

Iaspar Isac fecit 1635   Iacobus Theuart,   D. M. P.

3 b

CONSILIVM XCIII.

De Arthritide.

Morborvm quidam cogniti sunt, incogniti alij. Ad incognitos multa remedia adhibentur analogismo quodam & epilogismo quæsita, periculi faciundi causâ : & ita infra modum considetur, vt si non aliquod commemorabile auxiliū afferimus, saltem non obsimus. Et intereà si secundùm rationē

3c

De Ischiade.

CONSILIVM XCXV.

Dvos exercuêre dolores ischiadici, alij quidem oborti per humoris ἀπόθεσιν, sub finem febris longæ: alteri verò media

3d

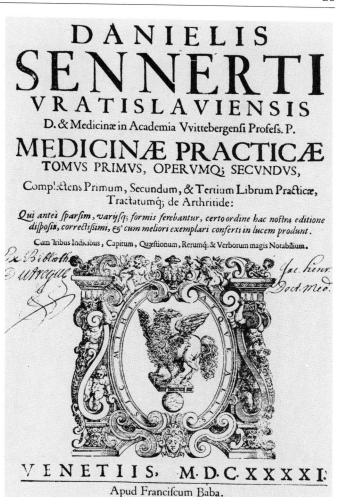

DANIELIS
SENNERTI
VRATISLAVIENSIS
D. & Medicinæ in Academia Vvittebergensi Profess. P.

MEDICINÆ PRACTICÆ
TOMVS PRIMVS, OPERVMQ; SECVNDVS,

Complectens Primum, Secundum, & Tertium Librum Practicæ,
Tractatumq; de Arthritide:

*Qui antea sparsim, varijsq; formis ferebantur, certo ordine hac nostra editione
dispositi, correctissimi, & cum meliori exemplari conferti in lucem produnt.*

Cum Tribus Indicibus, Capitum, Quæstionum, Rerumq. & Verborum magis Notabilium.

VENETIIS, M.DC.XXXXI.
Apud Franciscum Baba.
SVPERIORVM PERMISSV, ET PRIVILEGIO.

4a

Figs. **4a–e** The three volumes of the work "Medicinae practicae" by the physician *Daniel Sennert* of Breslau (1572–1637) was published in 1641 and included a chapter entitled "De Arthritide". Sennert, who still believed in pacts with the devil and in witches, distinguished between podagra, cheiragra, and gonagra, and when the hip is involved, sciatica. A play is devoted to the latter

24

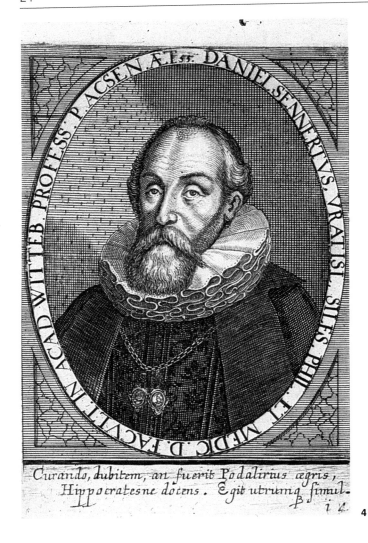

Curando, dubitem, an fuerit Podalirius ægris,
Hippocratesne docens. Egit utrumq; simul.

4b

condition (Fig. **4c, d**). The chapter on the catarrhs mentions the term "rheumatism" only once but it is not certain that he was referring to the modern concept of the disease.

860

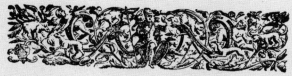

DE
ARTHRITIDE
TRACTATVS,

Appendicis loco Libro Tertio Practicæ adiectus.

CAPVT I.

De Natura Arthritidis.

Nomen.

RThritis, Græcis ἀπὸ τῦ ἄρθρυ, id est, articulo, dicta, Latinis morbus seu dolor articularis, à loco affecto nomen accepit. Barbari, quos ita vocant, Guttam appellant, quòd à fluxu quasi guttatim facto excitetur hoc malum. Et tunc ex recentioribus etiam, qui eos sequuntur, hanc appellationem omnibus præferunt, sed minus rectè, vt infra, quæst. 1. dicetur.

Αʹ;θωψ quid?

Etsi verò ἄρθων, vt ab Autore definit. Medicar.& Isagoges definitur, sit σύνδεσμ vel σύνθεσιν, compages & compositio ossium ad motum comparata: tamen hic per articulum non accipitur ipsa ossium compages, ac σύνδεσιν & vniò, vel extremitates ossium; quæ coniunguntur, vel spatium inter ossa, quæ articulo coniunguntur, sed partes, quæ ipsum articulum coniungunt & ambiunt, præcipuè sensu prædita, nimirùm, membranæ, ligamenta membranosa, & extremitates musculorum, partibusque his inserti nerui.

Arthritidis differentiæ pro varietate articulorum.

Cum verò articuli sint varii, ab eorum differentia, & varietate partium affectarum arthritis quoque varia nomina accepit, & si pedes afficiantur, dicitur Podagra, si manus, Chiragra; si coxendix, Ischias. si genu, Gonagra: vocabulis hisce plerisque à loco affecto & ἄγρα, quod capturam significat deducta, vt Podagra nihil aliud sit, quàm pedum, Chiragra verò manuum captura; cum hæc membra morbo hoc quasi capta & irretita detineantur: vnde etiam à Luciano, *in Tragopodagra*, sic loquens Podagra introducitur:

παρα δὶ τοῖς πεδίδις βροτῶν
πόδαγρα καλὶ μαι, γινομένη πεδῶν ἄγρα:

a plerisque autem hominum
Podagra vocor existens pedum captura.

In cæteris verò articulis speciale nomen non habet, sed communi generis nomine Arthritis appellatur; sicut & in genere Arthritis dicitur, cum plures articulos simul dolor occupat. Plura quidem talia vocabula finxerunt quidam & inter eos Ambrosius Parœus, *de arthrit. cap. 1.* & si malum in maxillæ articulo fuerit, Syagonagram; si in ceruice Trachelagram; si in spina dorsi, Rachysagram; si in humero Homagiam; si in cubito, Pechyagram nominant: Verùm vocabula ista apud

Græcos non occurrunt, nec vsu trita sunt; licet ipsi pluribus in partibus arthritidem generari posse passim doceant.

Mentagra quid?

Occurrit etiam apud Plinium, *lib.17 cap.1.* vocabulum Mentagræ, ioculari, vt Plinius ait, primum lasciuia inuentum (est enim vitiosa vocabuli con positio ex Latina & Græca voce, & aliena à consuetudine eruditorum) mox tamen vsurpatum: verùm affectus iste ad Arthritidem non pertinet, sed fuit faciei quædam fæditas, & praua scabies ad lichenes pertinens.

Græca vocabula & Latini retinuerunt, cùm ab iis & morbum acceperint. De quo Plinius, *lib. 26. c. 10.* Podagra, inquit, morbus rarior solebat esse non solùm patrum auorumque memoria, verùm & nostra, peregrinus & ipse. Nam si Italiæ fuisset antiquitus, Latinum nomen inuenisset.

Notandum tamen hic, etiamsi Podagræ vocabulum propriè de pedum dolore accipitur: tamen interdum, vt etiam Crato, *consil.253.* confitetur, ab vno membro desumpta appellatione pro omni arthritide podagra accipitur; cum fieri soleat, vt pedes ferè primò & frequentiùs hoc morbo corripiantur, & rarò cùm aliis articuli afficiuntur, immunes sint. Hinc quoque Dialogum suum, qui est de Arthritide, Lucianus Tragopodagram inscripsit. Ita qui de laude Podagræ scripserunt, Cardanus, & alii, omnes de Arthritide in genere egisse videntur; imò Medici quidà, qui propriè de arthritide agunt, tractatus suos de Podagra inscripserunt.

Arthritis quam lo-quentius inuadat?

Frequentius nimirùm pedes hic dolor, & quidem maximè ac primum ple rùnque pollicem pedis inuadit; Natura enim, quantum potest, humores vitiosos ad extrema & remotas partes depellere solet. funtq; pedes etiam à caloris fonte remotiores, & magis in motu, quo humores ad eos trahuntur. Vnde etiam Galenus, *6. aphor. 28.* scribit, eos, qui arthritide, id est, omnium articulorum doloribus corripiantur, primò fieri Podagricos. Vtplurimum verò hoc accidit, non verò semper. In quibusdam enim arthritis incipit in manu, quibusdam in genu, quibusdam in aliis articulis. Et quamuis primò pedes prehendit: tamè postea etiam frequentiùs in brachijs digitorum articulos, vel loca circa carpum & metacarpiũ occupat, vel & cubiti articulos inuadit, aliquando & cervix & maxillæ articulum. Et quidem malum hoc initio plerunque vnum articulum. vel in pede, quod frequentius accidit, vel alibi occupat, postea verò crebro morbi insultu visceribus debilitatis, ac calore natiuo labefactato, & materia indies magis cumulata, plures articulos inuadit, & res eo sæpe rediit,

PODAGRA TRAGICE
producta à Luciano.

Personæ colloquentes: Podager. Chorus Podagricorum. Podagra. Nuncius.
Duo Medici. Tortores.

Interprete M. ERASMO SCHMIDIO, Græc. & Math. Prof.

PODAGER.

O odiosum nomen, o Dijs inuisum,
Podagra planctibus abundans, Cocyti filia:
Quam Tartari latibulis in tenebrosissimis
Megæra Furia ventre edidit:
Vberibusq; enutriuit, & amarulento infanti
In labium instillauit lac Alecto.
Quisnam abominabilem te Dæmonum
In lucem produxit? Venisti hominibus noxa.
Si enim demortuos delictorum vltio
Homines sequitur, quæ patrarunt in vita:
Non Tantalum potibus (fugacibus,) neq; Ixionem
Rota versandum neq; Sisyphum saxo

Oportebat punire in domibus Plutonis:
Sed simpliciter omnes mala operatos
Tuis mancipare membra infestantibus doloribus.
Quam meum afflictum & miserum corpus
Manibus ab extremis in extremas pedum plantas,
Ichore malo, & amaro succo bilis,
Spiritu vehemente isto per stringens poros,
Effecit, & luctans intendit dolores:
Visceribusq; in ipsis ignitum discurrit Malum,
Vorticibus flammarum carnem ignis more depascens,
Veluti crater plenus Ætnæi ignis,
Aut † Siculus canalis æquorei interfluij.
Vbi confuse fluctuans
Ob fissuras petrarum obliquus voluitur æstus.

O cautu

4 d

De Catarrho.

Duo præcipuè vocabula occurrunt, quibus motus humorum præter naturam in corpore nostro exprimuntur. Generalissimum est ῥεῦμα & ῥευματισμὸς, fluxus seu fluxio, quæ vox omnem motum cuiuscunque humoris è quacunque in quamcunque partem nostri corporis significat. Κατάρροος καταρρ?ς, & καταρρος, Celso destillatio (malè enim Argenterium *in com. ad aphor.* 4. *libr.* 2. scripsisse, Latinos non habere proprium vocabulum, quo Catarrhi nomen exprimant, ex Plinio *libr.* 19. *cap.* 6. & *lib.* 23. *cap.* 8. patet) Græcis etiam aliàs κατασα-γμὸς tantum humoris superuacanei è capite & præcipuè cerebro in alias partes prolapsum & defluxum significant.

4 e

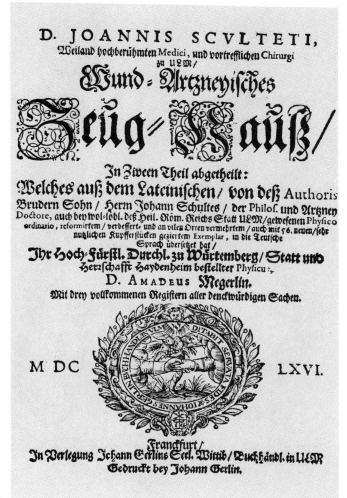

Figs. **5a** and **b** A book by the physician *Joannes Scultetus* (*Johann Schult-heiss*) of Ulm (1595–1646) was published in 1666, and it includes a figure of a female "with a fungous growth in the right knee".

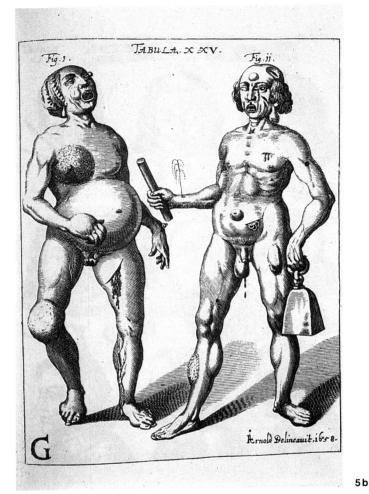

5b

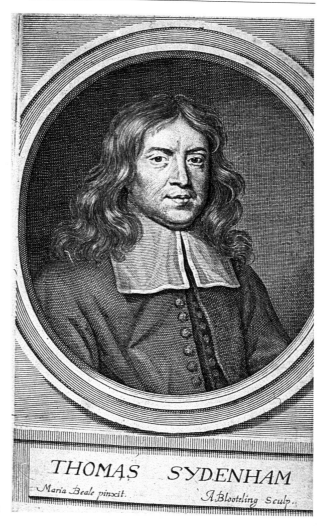

THOMAS SYDENHAM

Maria Beale pinxit. *A. Blooteling Sculp.*

6a

Figs. **6a–c** *Thomas Sydenham* (1624–1689) gave a detailed description of a gouty attack. He also differentiated gout from febrile acute and chronic rheumatism.

TRACTATUS

DE

Podagra

ET

HYDROPE.

PER

THO. SYDENHAM, M. D.

Non fingendum, aut excogitandum, fed
inveniendum, quid Natura faciat, aut
ferat. *Bacon.*

LONDINI, 1705.

6b

CAP. V.

Rheumatismus.

NUllo non tempore inceſſit hic morbus, maximè *Au-*
tumno, & præ cæteris annis florentes & οἷς γόνυ χλω-
ῷ. Hâc ut plurimùm occaſione naſcitur ; æger ſc.
ſîte exercitio aliquo vehementiori, ſive alio modo ex-
calefactus, mox repentinum frigus admiſit. A rigore
æque horrore orditur tragœdiam, quas ſtatim excipi-
unt calor, inquietudo, ſitis, & reliqua illa infelix ſym-
ptomatum caterva, quibus ſtipantur Febres. Elapſo
die uno alterove, (eſt & ubi citiùs) æger atroci dolore,
nunc in hoc, nunc in illo artu infeſtatur, in carpis,
humeris, genubus præſertim ; qui locum ſubinde mu-
tans, viciſſim illos occupat, rubore quodam & tumore
a parte quam poſtremùm affecit adhuc reſiduis. Pri-
ris aliquot diebus, Febris & ſymptomata jam memo-
rata quandoque coincidunt ; Febris autem ſenſim eva-
nidit, manente dolore, quin & nonnunquam immani-
us ſæviente, materiâ ſc. febrili in artus translatâ ; quod.
ſatis arguit Febris ipſa ſæpiùs recrudeſcens ob mate-
riam morbificam ab intempeſtivo Externorum uſu re-
percuſſam. Morbus hic quoties à Febre ſejungitur, *Ar-*
thritis ſæpe audit ; quamvis eſſentialiter ab illâ diſtin-
guatur, prout cuivis facilè conſtabit, cui uterque morbus intimiùs fuerit perſpectus : unde forſan petenda
à ratio, cur tam ſicco illum pede tranſiverint ſcrip-
tores Medici : Niſi forte arbitremur, hanc morbi ſpe-
ciem ad reliquam malorum Iliada de novo acceſſiſſe.
Unt ſe res habeat, jam plus ſatis graſſatur hic morbus ; & licèt rariſſimè hominem è medio tollat, Febre
ſemel depulſâ, tamen & vehementia doloris & diutur-
nitas eum prorſus contemni non ſinunt. Etenim ſi
etiam peritè tractetur, non ad menſes tantùm, ſed ad
annos etiam aliquot, imò per omnem adeò vitam mi-
ſerum

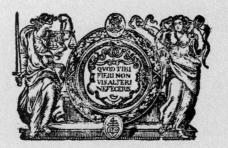

GUILHELMI

MUSGRAVE

M. D. Inclyti Medicorum Londinenſium Collegii,
& Regiæ Societatis Socii,

DE

ARTHRITIDE

SYMPTOMATICA

DISSERTATIO.

Αγαθοῖσι δὲ Ἰητροῖσιν αἱ Ὁμοιότητες πλάνας καὶ ἀπορείας. *Hippocr.*

EDITIO NOVA *accuratior.*

QVOD TIBI
FIERI NON
VIS ALTERI
NE FECERIS

GENEVÆ.
Apud FRATRES DE TOURNES.

M. DCCXV.

7a

Figs. **7a–d** In 1715 the English physician *William Musgrave* (1655–1721) of Exeter published several works on arthritic disorders of varied origin.

ELENCHUS.

7b

GUILHELMI

MUSGRAVE

M. D. Inclyti Medicorum Londinensium Collegii,
& Regiæ Societatis Socii,

D E

ARTHRITIDE

ANOMALA, SIVE INTERNA,

DISSERTATIO.

Καὶ τῦτο δ᾽ εἰδέναι χρὴ, εἴτε Λύει ἢ Νᾶσος, εἴτε Μεταπίπτει ἐς ἐτέρκ Νᾶσον. *Hippocr.*

E D I T I O N O V A *accuratior.*

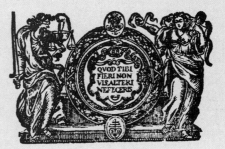

QVOD TIBI
FIERI NON
VIS ALTERI
NE FECERIS

G E N E V Æ.

Apud FRATRES DE TOURNES.

M. DCCXV.

7c

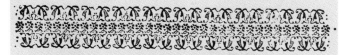

ELENCHUS.

DE

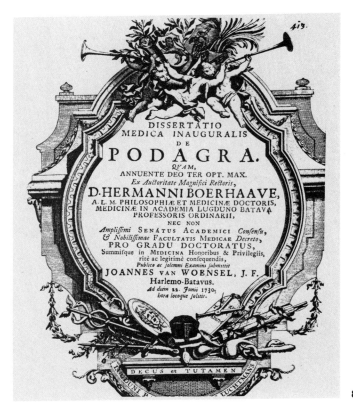

413.

DISSERTATIO
MEDICA INAUGURALIS
DE
PODAGRA.
QVAM,
ANNUENTE DEO TER OPT. MAX.
Ex Auctoritate Magnifici Rectoris,
D·HERMANNI BOERHAAVE,
A. L. M. PHILOSOPHIÆ ET MEDICINÆ DOCTORIS,
MEDICINÆ IN ACADEMIA LUGDUNO BATAVA
PROFESSORIS ORDINARII,
NEC NON
Amplissimi SENATUS ACADEMICI *Consensu,*
& *Nobilissimae* FACULTATIS MEDICAE *Decreto,*
PRO GRADU DOCTORATUS,
Summisque in MEDICINA Honoribus & Privilegiis,
ritè ac legitimè consequendis,
Publico ac solemni Examinis submittit
JOANNES van WOENSEL, J. F.
Harlemo-Batavus.
Ad diem 22. *Junii* 1730.
hora locoque solitis.

DECUS et TUTAMEN

8a

Figs. **8a** and **b**   *Hermann Boerhaave* (1668–1738), was a professor at Leiden, and became a teacher of international fame (his disciples were, among others, *Cullen*, Haller, and *van Swieten*). His having gout was probably the impetus for a thesis on podagra written by one of his pupils.

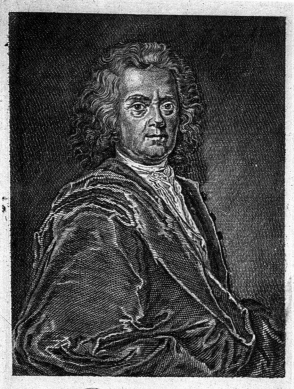

Hermann Boerhave

Wandelaar del.   Hauke Sculps.

8 b

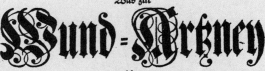

D. LAURENTII Heisters,

Braunschweig-Lüneburgischer Hof-Rath und Leib-Medicus, Medicinæ,
Chirurgiæ und Botanices Professor auf der Königl. und Hertzogl. Julius-Universität zu
Helmstädt, auch Mitglied der Käyserlichen, Königlichen Englischen
und Preußischen Societät.

CHIRURGIE,

In welcher alles,
Was zur

Wund-Artzney

gehöret,

Nach der neuesten und besten Art, gründlich abgehandelt,
und in Acht und dreyßig Kupffer-Tafeln
die neu-erfundene und dienlichste

Instrumente,

Nebst den bequemsten Handgriffen der Chirurgischen
Operationen und Bandagen
deutlich vorgestellet werden.

Neue viel vermehrte und verbesserte Auflage.

Mit Röm. Kayserl. wie auch Königl. Pohln. und Churfürstl. Sächß. allergnädigst. PRIVILEGIIS.

Nürnberg,
Bey Johann Adam Stein, und Gabriel Nicolaus Raspe, 1752.

9 a

Figs. **9a–c** *Lorenz Heister* (1683–1758), the founder of scientific surgery (including anatomy) in Germany described "fungus of the limbs and dropsy of the joints" (probably meaning synovitis). However it is unknown whether the synovitis was a manifestation of rheumatoid arthritis or of tuberculosis.

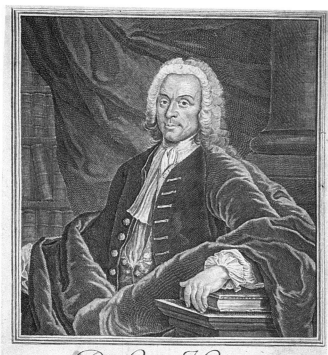

9b

D. Laur. Heister
Medicinæ Chir. ac Botanices
Prof. Publ. Helmstad.

Das 19. Capitel.
Vom Glied-Schwamm und Wassersucht in den Gelencken.

I.

Was ein Glied-Schwamm sey.

Zu den wässerigen Geschwülsten kommen sehr nahe die sogenannten Glied-Schwämme: welche sehr beschwerliche und offt übel zu curirende Geschwülste an den Gelencken sind, aber von vielen Auctoren mit Stillschweigen übergangen, von andern aber obenhin tractiret oder berühret werden: vielleicht deßwegen, weil die meisten nicht gewußt, ob selbige Geschwülste vom Geblüte, Gewässer, Materie, Winden oder andern widernatürlichen Ursachen entstanden oder zu entstehen pflegen. Es sind aber die Glied-Schwämme lake und bleiche Geschwülste an den Gelencken, weichlich und fast wie ein Schwamm anzufühlen; welche aber vom Eindrücken keine Gruben behalten, auch wenig oder gar keinen Schmertzen verursachen, dennoch die Bewegung und Gebrauch des Gelencks verhindern: als woran man diese Geschwülste erkennen, und von andern unterscheiden kan. Sie entstehen wohl an allerley Gelencken der Arme und Beine, am öfftersten aber an den Knien: welches daher zu geschehen scheinet, weil außher in dem Gelencke ziemliche Drüsen, auch zwischen den Ligamenten und Flechsen vieles Fett lieget; dieses Gelencke auch bey vielen und Stossen vielen Verletzungen unterworffen: daher sich gerne allerley Feuchtigkeiten hier zu stocken und zu sammlen pflegen. Zuweilen stecken diese Feuchtigkeiten ausser dem Gelencke, welches eigentlich ein Glied-Schwamm; manchmal aber in dem Gelencke selbsten, welches eine Wassersucht des Gelenckes kan genannt werden. Diese erkennet man aus einer Geschwulst, welche das gantze Glied fast gleich dicke machet; jener aber ist mehr auf einer Seite. Es sind selbige manchmal sehr groß; einmal weicher, das andermal härter anzufühlen: welches von der daselbst stockenden flüßigern oder dickern Feuchtigkeit zu entstehen pfleget *a).*

Ursache.

2. Die nächste Ursache der Glied-Schwämme ist eine Stockung und Versammlung eines zähen, schleimigen Gewässers zwischen der Haut, und entweder

a) Ein sehr grosser Glied-Schwamm ist abgebildet zu sehen in Purmanns Chirurgia curiosa pag. 622.

9c

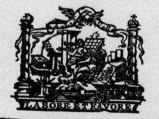

ANTONII STÖRCK,

SACRÆ CÆSAR. REG. APOST. MAJESTATIS· CONSILIARII AULICI,
ARCHIATRI, ET IN NOSOCOMIO CIVICO PAZMARIANO PHYSICI,

ANNUS MEDICUS
SECUNDUS,

QUO SISTUNTUR

OBSERVATIONES

CIRCA

MORBOS ACUTOS ET CHRONICOS,

ADJICIUNTURQUE

EORUM CURATIONES,

ET QUÆDAM

ANATOMICÆ CADAVERUM
SECTIONES.

EDITIO ALTERA.

VINDOBONÆ,

TYPIS JOANNIS THOMÆ TRATTNER, CÆS. REG.
MAJEST. AULÆ TYPOGRAPHI.

MDCCLXII.

10a

Figs. **10a–c** In 1762, Baron *Anton von Störck* (1731–1803), personal physician to the empress Maria Theresa, published a book with a chapter "De febre continua arthritica aut rheumatica." He suggested the influence of climate on arthritic or rheumatic fever. He was the first in Europe to use the plant Colchicum for the treatment of gout.

De febre continua arthritica, &
rheumatica.

Autumno, hyeme, & vere multi aderant in nosocomio, qui febre continua arthritica, aut rheumatica laborarunt.

Aër humidus, nebulosus, & frigidus hos morbos plerumque produxit.

In principio horror & frigus spinam dorsi, aut integrum quandoque corpus permearunt; dein orta est febris & sitis, & mox prodiit urina crassa, jumentosa.

Post aliquot horas accessit dolor vagus, qui
eodem

10b

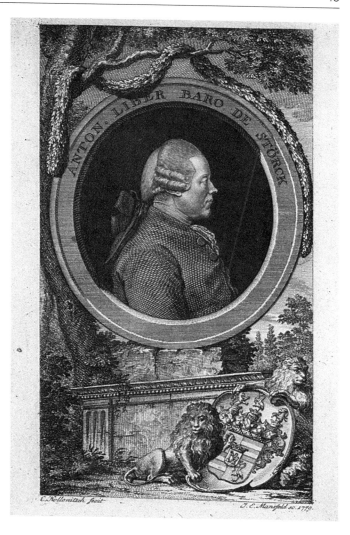

ANTON. LIBER BARO DE STÖRCK.

C. Kollonitsch fecit

J. E. Mansfeld sc. 1779.

10c

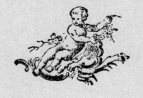

Joseph Jakob Plenks,

der Chirurgie Doktor, der Wundarzney, Anatomie und
Entbindungskunst ordentlichen Lehrer auf der königlichen Universität zu Ofen,

Anfangsgründe

der

Chirurgie.

Für

die angehenden Wundärzte

im

Königreich Hungarn.

Pest,
in der Weingand = und Köpfischen Buchhandlung.
1783.

11 a

Figs. **11 a–b** In the book by *Josef Jakob Plenk* (1732–1807) the brief definition of "fungous disease of the limbs" probably was not based on pathologic-anatomic studies.

Der Gliedschwamm.

Ist eine Geschwulst, deren enthaltenes Wesen eine schwammichte Fetthaut ist.

Der gewöhnlichste Sitz dieser Geschwulst ist am Kniegelenke, oder am Elbogen.

Die Heilung. Sie läßt sich oft durch das Gliedschwammpflaster zertheilen.

11 b

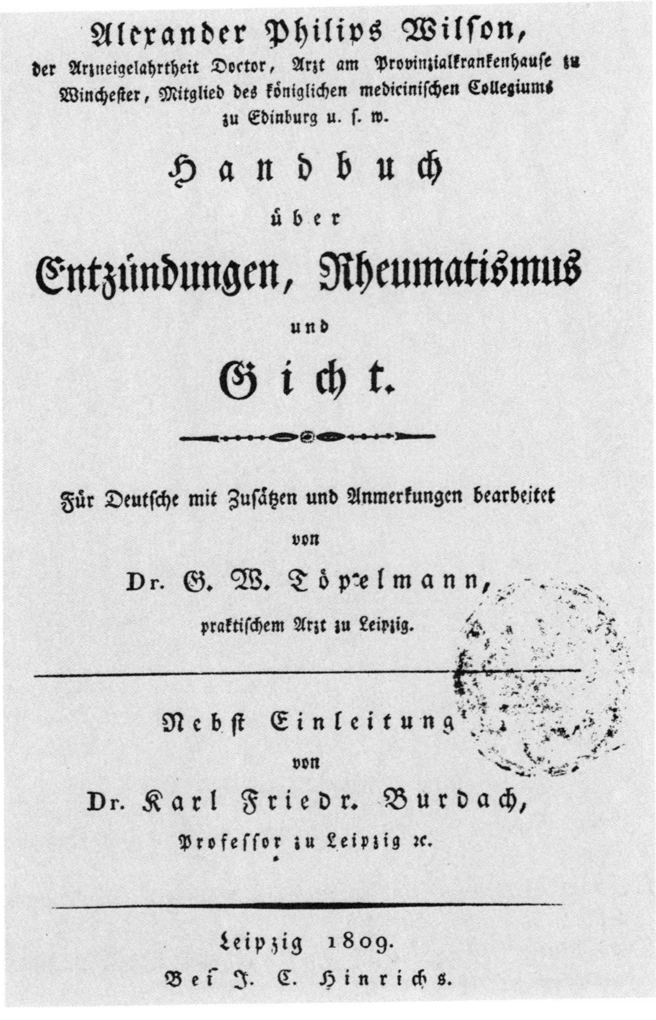

Alexander Philips Wilson,

der Arzneigelahrtheit Doctor, Arzt am Provinzialkrankenhause zu
Winchester, Mitglied des königlichen medicinischen Collegiums
zu Edinburg u. s. w.

Handbuch

über

Entzündungen, Rheumatismus

und

Gicht.

Für Deutsche mit Zusätzen und Anmerkungen bearbeitet

von

Dr. G. W. Töpelmann,

praktischem Arzt zu Leipzig.

Nebst Einleitung

von

Dr. Karl Friedr. Burdach,

Professor zu Leipzig ꝛc.

Leipzig 1809.

Bei J. C. Hinrichs.

12a

Figs. **12a–d** In the translation of a book by *Alexander Philips Wilson*, also called *A. W. Philip,* with an introduction by *K. F. Burdach* (1776–1847), the discoverer of the fasciculus cuneatus of Burdach in the spinal cord, "rheumatism" is differentiated from "gout" according to *William Cullen* (1712–1790). (Fig. **12d** reproduced from *F. H. Garrison:* An Introduction to the History of Medicine. Saunders, Philadelphia 1913.)

Neuntes Kapitel.

Rheumatismus.

Der Rheumatismus ist, gleich der Hepatitis, entweder hitziger oder chronischer Art. Von der letztern Form werde ich nur weniges sagen, weil sie eigentlich nicht zu der Klasse fieberhafter Entzündungen gehört. Dieß ist zwar auch mit der chronischen Leberentzündung der Fall; allein, da diese Krankheit mehr zu bedeuten hat, und weit weniger einfach als der chronische Rheumatismus ist, auch hin und wieder von mehr oder weniger Fieber begleitet wird, so glaubte ich, hiermit eine Ausnahme machen zu können.

Cullen bestimmt den hitzigen Rheumatismus als eine Krankheit, die durch eine äußerliche und meistentheils deutlich zu erkennende Ursache erregt wird, mit Fieber und Schmerz in den Gelenken, welcher bei äußerer Wärme zunimmt, in die muskulösen Theile schießt, und die Kniee nebst andern größern Gelenken mehr als die kleinern an den Händen und Füßen befällt.

Der erste Theil dieser Definition leidet Einwürfe. Die Ursachen einer Krankheit dürfen nie in einen nosologischen Charakter eingeführt werden, sie müssen denn in vorzüglichem Grade einleuchten und die diagnostischen Symptome

Zehntes Kapitel.

Von der Gicht.

Cullen bestimmt den hitzigen Rheumatismus als eine Krankheit, die durch eine äußerliche und meistentheils deutlich zu erkennende Ursache erregt wird, mit Fieber und Schmerz in den Gelenken, welcher bei äußerer Wärme zunimmt, in die muskulösen Theile schießt, und die Kniee nebst andern größern Gelenken mehr als die kleinern an den Händen und Füßen befällt.

Cullen bestimmt die Gicht als eine erbliche Krankheit, die ohne eine äußerliche, in die Sinne fallende Ursache entsteht, aber meistentheils ungewöhnliche Beschwerden des Magens zum Vorgänger hat, mit Fieber und Schmerz in den Gelenken verbunden ist, welcher letztere am häufigsten die Gelenke der Hand und des Fußes, insonderheit die der großen Zehe befällt, von Zeit zu Zeit wieder kommt, und oft mit Affektion des Magens oder anderer innern Theile abwechselt.

12c

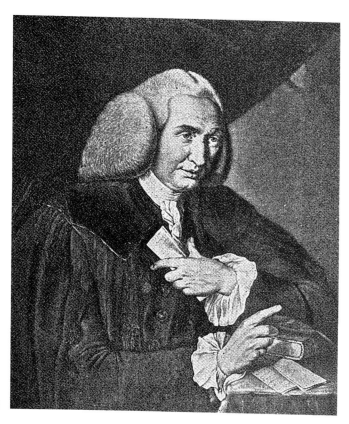

12 d

GULIELMI HEBERDEN

COMMENTARII

DE

MORBORUM HISTORIA

ET

CURATIONE.

RECUDI CURAVIT

S. TH. SOEMMERRING.

Γέρων, καὶ κάμπτειν οὐκέτι δυνάμενος, τοῦτο τὸ βιβλίον ἔγραψα, συντάξας τὰς μετὰ πολλῆς τριβῆς ἐν ταῖς τῶν ἀνθρώπων νόσοις καταληφθεί- σας μοι πείρας.

ALEX. TRALL. Lib. XII.

FRANCOFURTI AD MOENUM
APUD VARRENTRAPP ET WENNER
MDCCCIV.

13a

Figs. **13a–b** *William Heberden* (1710–1801), here quoted by the distin- guished physician, anatomist, and scientist *S. Th. Soemmering*, described the nodes over the dorsal aspects of the distal interphalangeal joints, which were named after him. He already recognized that these nodes are not a manifesta- tion of gout, although even today the lay public terms them "gouty nodes", and

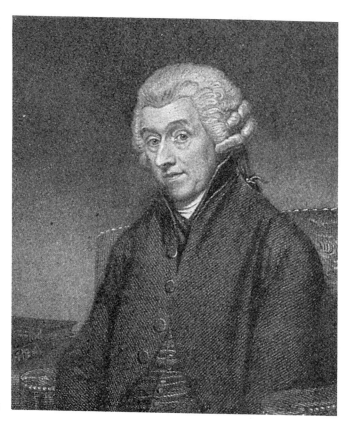

13b

they are even classified among rheumatoid arthritis. (Fig. **13b** reproduced from *F. H. Garrison*: An Introduction to the History of Medicine. Saunders, Philadelphia 1913.)

TRAITÉ

SUR LA NATURE ET LE TRAITEMENT

DE LA GOUTTE
ET DU RHUMATISME,

Renfermant des Considérations générales sur l'état morbide des organes digestifs, des Remarques sur le régime, et des Observations pratiques sur la gravelle;

Par Charles SCUDAMORE.

Traduit de l'anglais sur la dernière édition, par C. F.

DEUXIÈME ÉDITION,

Augmentée, 1° d'une Addition contenant les principes de la nouvelle Doctrine médicale de M. Broussais, sur la Goutte, par M. Goupil, Docteur en Médecine; 2° d'un Mémoire sur l'emploi des Bains de Vapeur dans les affections rhumatismales, par un Médecin de l'hôpital Saint-Louis;

AVEC DES PLANCHES REPRÉSENTANT TOUS LES APPAREILS EMPLOYÉS DANS CET HÔPITAL.

TOME PREMIER.

PARIS,
CHEZ BÉCHET JEUNE,
LIBRAIRE DE L'ACADÉMIE ROYALE DE MÉDECINE,
place de l'École de Médecine, n° 4.

1823.

14

Fig. **14** In 1823 *Charles Scudamore* described rheumatism and gout, making use of chemical urinalysis, in diagnosis.

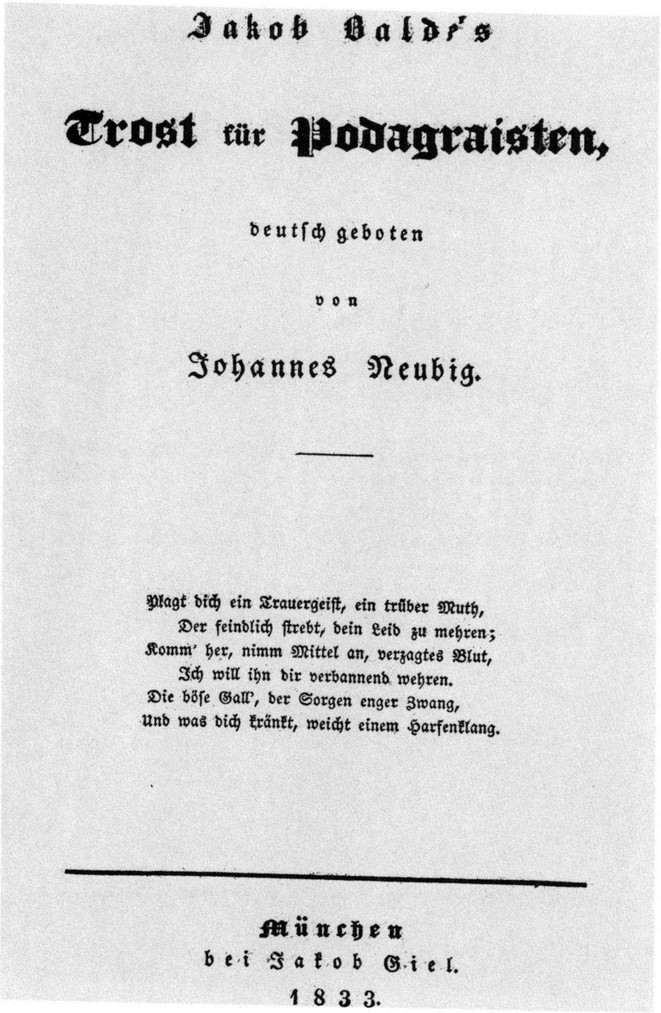

Jakob Balde's

Trost für Podagraisten,

deutsch geboten

von

Johannes Neubig.

———

Plagt dich ein Trauergeist, ein trüber Muth,
Der feindlich strebt, dein Leid zu mehren;
Komm' her, nimm Mittel an, verzagtes Blut,
Ich will ihn dir verbannend wehren.
Die böse Gall', der Sorgen enger Zwang,
Und was dich kränkt, weicht einem Harfenklang.

———

München
bei Jakob Giel.
1 8 3 3.

15

Fig. **15** This booklet published in 1833, which today makes a curious impression, was intended for the tormented patient with gout.

Neue Untersuchungen

über den

acuten Rheumatismus

der Gelenke

im Allgemeinen,

und

über das Gesetz

der Coincidenz der Pericarditis und Endocarditis

mit demselben im Besondern

so wie auch

über die Wirksamkeit der rasch auf einander folgenden Blutentziehungen bei dessen Behandlung

vom

Professor Dr. Bouillaud.

Aus dem Französischen

vom

Dr. Kersten.

His observatis, nemo rationis capax jure in his morbis vituperare missionem sanguinis potest, sed mirifice et tanquam divinum auxilium commendare, extollere et confidenter usurpare.
Botalli: De Curatione per venae - sectionem.

Magdeburg,

Verlag von Eduard Bühler.

1837.

16a

Figs. **16a–b** *Jean-Baptiste Bouillaud* (1796–1881) recognized the close relationship between rheumatic fever and endocarditis. The disease has become a rarity in the antibiotic era. (Fig. **16b** reproduced from *F. H. Garrison*: An Introduction to the History of Medicine. Saunders, Philadelphia 1913.)

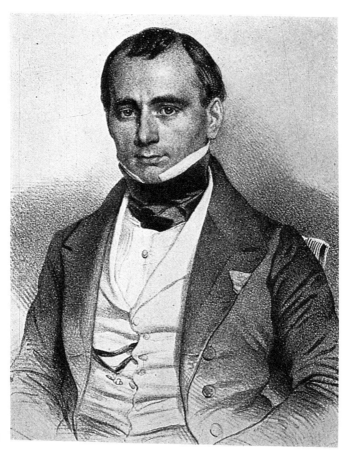

16 b

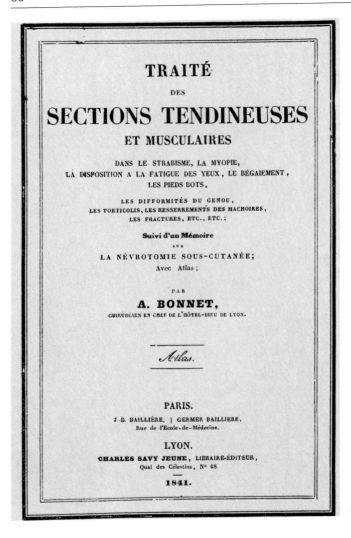

17 a

Figs. **17a–c** *Amédée Bonnet* of Lyon (1802–1888) described lesions that can be definitely regarded as the result of rheumatoid arthritis. He also proposed the division of tendons and muscles to promote motion in contractures of joints. (Fig. **17c** reproduced from *B. Valentin*: Geschichte der Orthopädie. Thieme, Stuttgart 1961.)

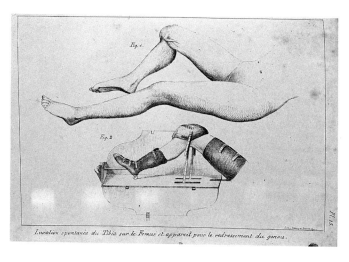

Fig. 1.

Fig. 2

Luxation spontanée du Tibia sur le Femur et appareil pour le redressement du genou.

Pl. 15.

17 b

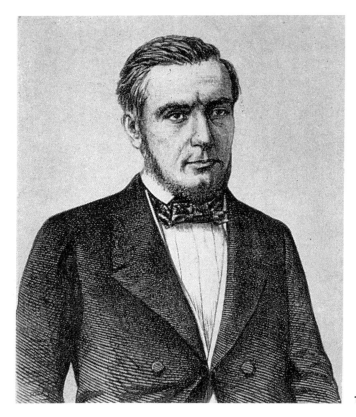

17c

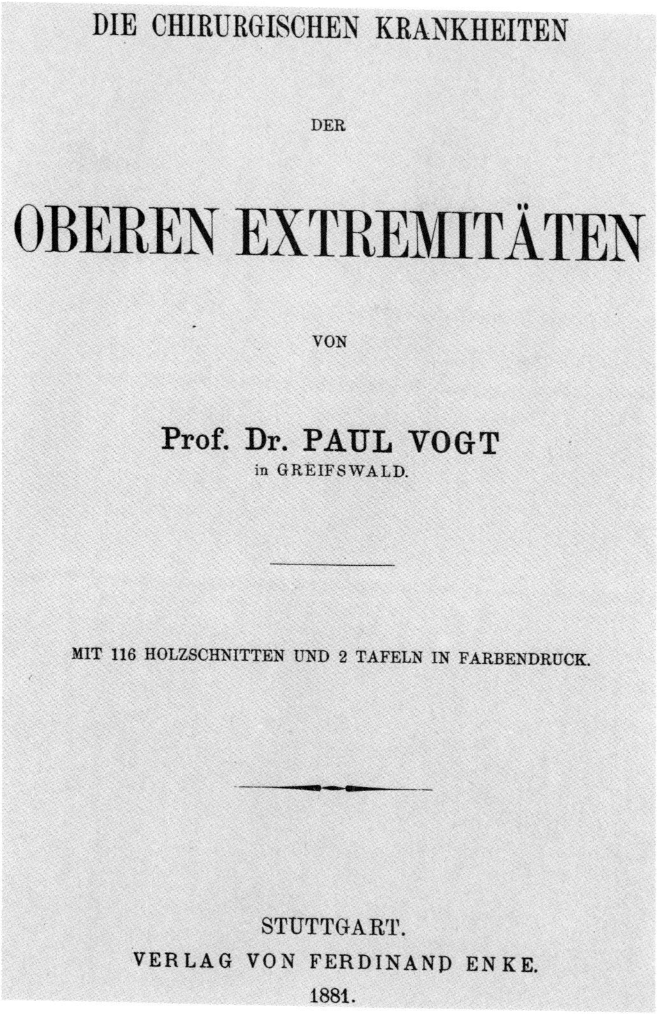

DIE CHIRURGISCHEN KRANKHEITEN

DER

OBEREN EXTREMITÄTEN

VON

Prof. Dr. PAUL VOGT

in GREIFSWALD.

MIT 116 HOLZSCHNITTEN UND 2 TAFELN IN FARBENDRUCK.

STUTTGART.

VERLAG VON FERDINAND ENKE.

1881.

18a

Figs. **18a–d** A monograph by *Paul Vogt* described conspicuous rheumatic lesions. This writer illustrated marked multiple tophi at the olecranon bursa in gout and also tophi distributed over the entire hand (probably borrowed from *Alfred Garrod* [1859]). Other illustrations show a swan-neck deformity in the hand, a typical sequel of rheumatoid arthritis, here erroneously termed "gouty affection of the finger", as well as a massive bursitis in the shoulder region.

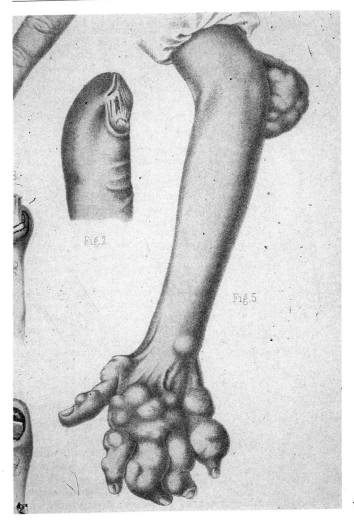

Fig.2.

Fig.5

18b

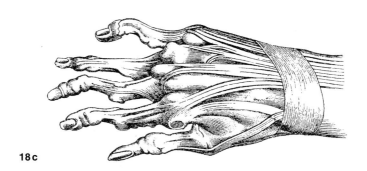

18 c

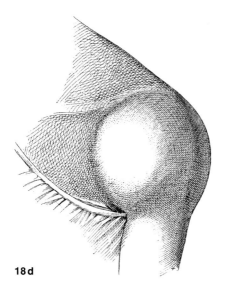

18 d

MALADIES

PAR

RALENTISSEMENT

DE LA NUTRITION

COURS DE PATHOLOGIE GÉNÉRALE

PROFESSÉ A LA FACULTÉ DE MÉDECINE DE PARIS
PENDANT L'ANNÉE 1879-1880

Par Ch. BOUCHARD

Professeur de Pathologie et de Thérapeutique générales
Médecin des Hôpitaux

RECUEILLI ET PUBLIÉ

PAR LE Dʳ H. FRÉMY

PARIS

LIBRAIRIE F. SAVY

77, BOULEVARD SAINT-GERMAIN, 77

—

1882

19a

Figs. **19a–b** In 1882, *Charles Bouchard* pointed out in his book entitled *"Maladies par Ralentissoment de la Nutrition"* the supposed relationships between rheumatic changes and disorders of the gastrointestinal tract. He also presumed relationships between a past infection and rheumatoid arthritis. It is possible that he failed to differentiate the osteoarthritis of the proximal interphalangeal joints named after him.

TRENTIÈME LEÇON.

PATHOGÉNIE DU RHUMATISME ARTICULAIRE AIGU.

Affinités pathologiques du rhumatisme. Rapports du rhumatisme musculaire, du rhumatisme articulaire et du rhumatisme articulaire chronique avec la lithiase biliaire, l'obésité, le diabète et la goutte. — Les maladies rhumatismales forment une famille morbide dans la tribu des maladies par nutrition retardante.

Le rhumatisme articulaire aigu. — Etiologie. Distribution géographique. Races. Saisons. Épidémies rhumatiques. Ages. Sexe. Professions. Retour des accès. Hérédité. Refroidissement. Secousses morales. Chocs traumatiques.

Pathogénie. Théorie embolique. Théorie infectieuse. Théorie névrotrophique. Théorie humorale.

19b

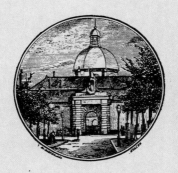

OEUVRES COMPLÈTES

DE

J. M. CHARCOT

MALADIES DES VIEILLARDS
GOUTTE ET RHUMATISME

TOME VII

AVEC 19 FIGURES DANS LE TEXTE ET 4 PLANCHES

PARIS

AUX BUREAUX DU PROGRÈS MÉDICAL | LECROSNIER ET BABÉ
14, rue des Carmes. | LIBRAIRES-ÉDITEURS
| Place de l'École-de-Médecine.

1889

Tous droits réservés.

20a

Figs. **20a–e** The neurologist *Jean-Martin Chargot* (1825–1893) possibly described rheumatoid arthritis as early as 1853. It is, however, certain that in 1889 he presented a detailed description of this disease. He differentiated among other lesions the deformities of the fingers that later were termed "swan-neck" and "buttonhole" deformities. The impressive figures in his book,

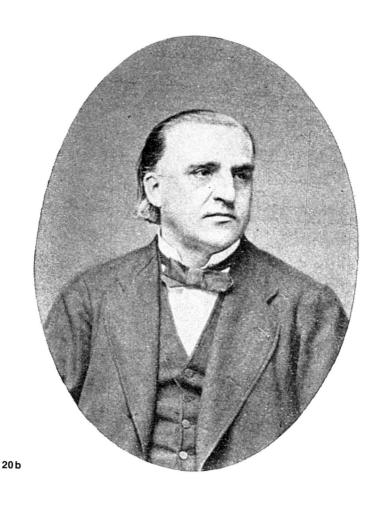

20 b

especially those of the hand, allow discriminating between degenerative and inflammatory disorders. The characteristics of gout are also appreciated. (Fig. **20 b** reproduced from *F. H. Garrison:* An Introduction to the History of Medicine. Saunders, Philadelphia 1913.)

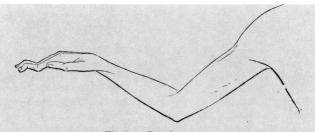

Fig. 9. — Premier type.

Ce type peut offrir deux variétés. Dans la première, la plupart des caractères que nous avons décrits sont conservés ; seulement la phalangine et la phalange sont sur le même axe, et forment une seule colonne.

20 c

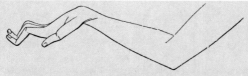

Fig. 12. — Second type.

Ce type peut offrir, comme le précédent, deux variétés.
Dans la première, il y a flexion de toutes les articulations de la main les unes sur les autres, de manière à constituer une sorte d'enroulement.

20 d

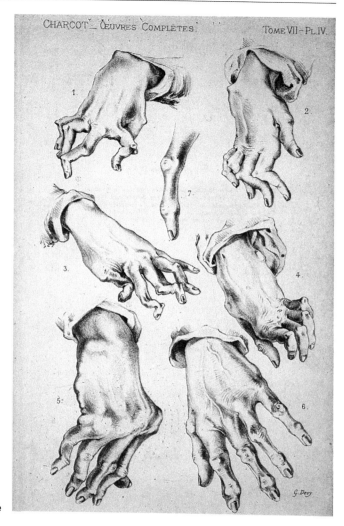

CHARCOT — Œuvres Complètes.

Tome VII — Pl. IV.

G. Devy

20 e

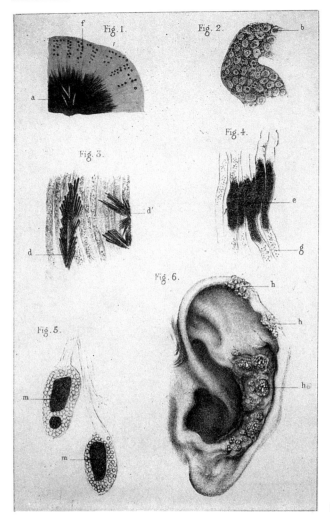

Fig. 1.
Fig. 2.
Fig. 3.
Fig. 4.
Fig. 5.
Fig. 6.

20f

Clinical Pictures

Rheumatoid Arthritis

Rheumatoid arthritis is a systemic disease of frequent occurrence that runs a variable episodic course. It is chiefly characterized by inflammation of the synovial tissues in isolated or numerous joints, tendon sheaths, and bursae, as well as by humoral signs of inflammation. Occasionally, in favorable cases, it can heal at a relatively early stage without sequelae. In numerous unfavorable instances, however, it leads to destruction or ankylosis of joints, so that the patient even may become bedridden and, dependent on help from others. Internal organs can become involved. There exist numerous subtypes of the disease. Rheumatoid arthritis is seldom fatal.

Articular Synovitis, Tenosynovitis, and their Sequelae in the Upper Extremities

Shoulder

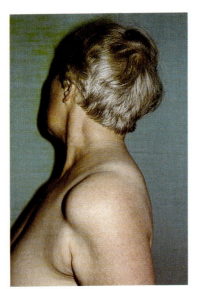

1

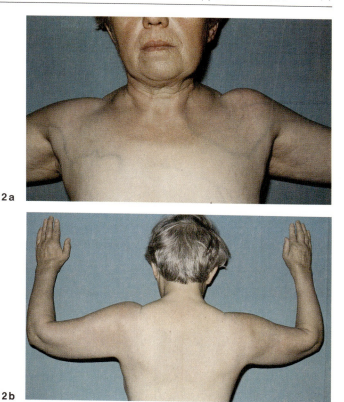

2a

2b

Fig. **1** Rheumatoid arthritis with synovitis of the left shoulder joint with involvement of the subdeltoid bursa, in a 60-year-old female. Marked swelling can be seen, particularly in the anterior and less in the superior portion of the shoulder joint.

Figs. **2a** and **b** With diminished abduction of the right arm at the shoulder joint because of painful synovitis, the shoulder itself is concomitantly raised and adducted.

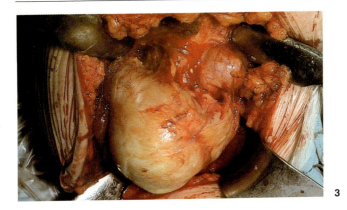

3

Fig. 3 Shown is the markedly enlarged subdeltoid bursa that communicates with the shoulder joint. Above right: capsule of the shoulder joint.

Fig. 4 Deposition of fibrin in the bursa in the form of rice bodies. The superjacent synovial capsule of the shoulder joint itself, which is markedly widened and thickened, has not yet been opened.

4   **6**

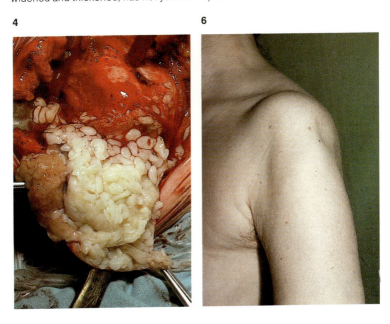

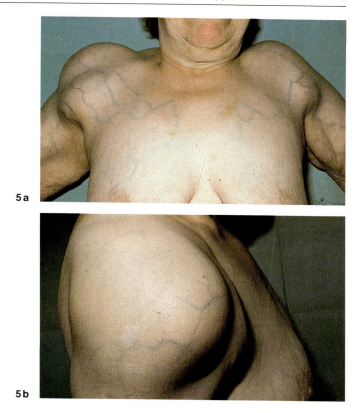

5a

5b

Figs. **5a** and **b**   Extreme synovitis of both shoulder joints with involvement of the adjacent bursae. The figure shows the maximal possible abduction at both shoulder joints. On attempting abduction, both shoulders are concomitantly raised. The movements in all other directions are also restricted as a result of the marked synovitis and the advanced changes in the glenoid and the head of the humerus. This is a 55-year-old female with rheumatoid arthritis with advanced changes in numerous joints and resulting considerable limitation of movement.

Fig. **6**   43-year-old female with active rheumatoid arthritis. Massive synovitis in numerous joints. The restriction of motion in the left shoulder joint produced by the inflammation has led to atrophy of the entire deltoid muscle. The arthritic lesions of the shoulder joint and the muscular atrophy are the cause of considerable limitation of motion.

Shoulder Girdle

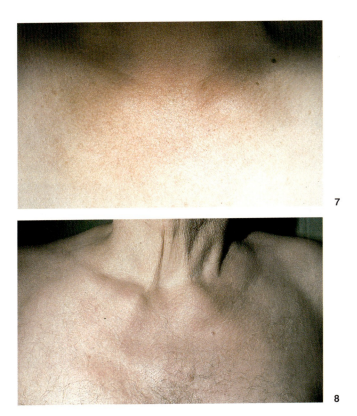

7

8

Fig. **7**   Involvement of the sternoclavicular joints in rheumatic arthritis can give rise to discomfort on moving the head, the shoulder girdle, and even the thorax. The patient complains of oppression, and occasionally of apprehension, on breathing and swallowing. Synovitis of the sternoclavicular joint is more marked on the left than on the right side.

Fig. **8**   Advanced lesions of synovitis in the left sternoclavicular joint of a 67-year-old female with rheumatoid arthritis.

Figs. **9a** and **b**   Synovitis of the elbow joint with distention of the radial compartment of the joint in the vicinity of the head of the radius.

Elbow Joint

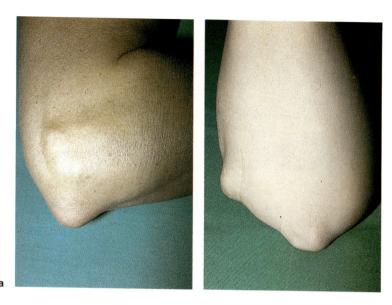

a   9 b

Fig. **10** Marked synovitis with swelling over the head of the radius. The swelling can be pushed into the joint by finger pressure. When the examiner places a thumb on the head of the radius and rotates the right-angled arm at the elbow joint, the palpable crepitation allows diagnosing an even slight synovitis of the elbow joint.

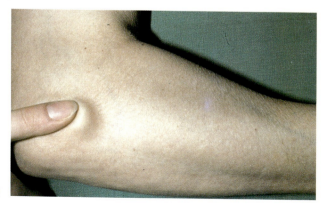

10

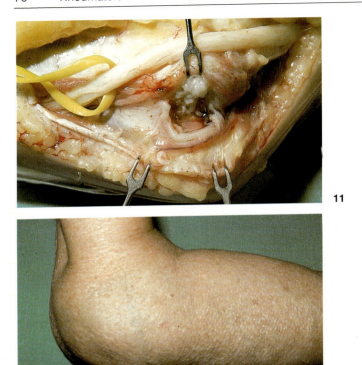

11

12

Fig. **11** Elbow joint opened for synovectomy through the medial olecranon groove. There exists a synovitis with fibrin deposits. The pocketing of the joint in the groove can give rise to ulnar nerve compression with the corresponding neurologic deficits in the lower arm and, especially, the hand. After decompression and neurolysis, the nerve is translocated into the antecubital fossa.

Fig. **12** Monstrous synovitis of the right elbow joint. In contrast, the entire musculature of the upper arm is markedly atrophic.

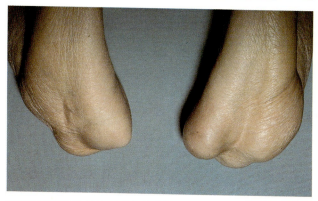

13a

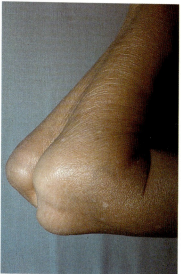

13b

Figs. **13a** and **b**   Deformation of both elbow joints and the proximal lower arms as the result of the disease process. The total instability of the joint allows full flexion.

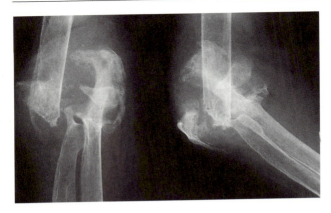

14

Fig. **14**   Comminuted fracture of the right elbow joint in extreme deformity (Roentgenograms in two planes).

Figs. **15a** and **b**   Completely unstable elbow joint as the result of the disease process. When the upper arm is fixed, maximal radial and ulnar abduction can be performed.

15a

15b

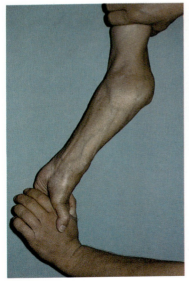

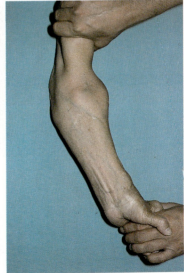

Hand

Articular Synovitis and its Consequences

Wrist

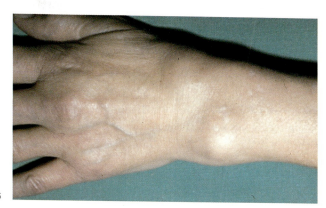

16

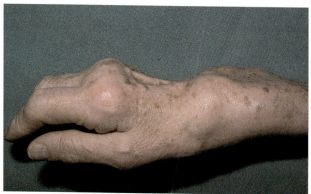

17

Fig. **16** 44-year-old female with rheumatoid arthritis. Swelling of the wrist in the vicinity of the head of the ulna and in the radial compartment of the joint from articular synovitis. The swelling extends to the radial intercarpal region. Synovitis of the third metacarpophalangeal joint.

Fig. **17** Articular synovitis of the radial and ulnar regions of the wrist, associated with tenosynovitis of the radial and ulnar extensor tendons in a 68-year-old female. Involvement of the metacarpophalangeal joints

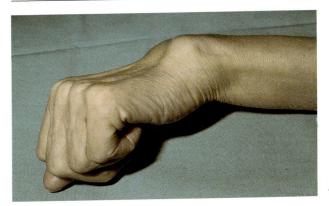

Fig. **18** Instability with volar dislocation of the entire wrist as the result of articular synovitis in a 62-year-old female.

Metacarpophalangeal joint

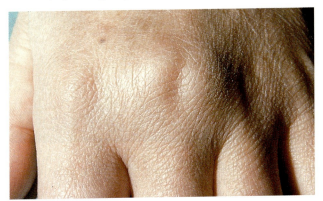

Fig. **19** 52-year-old female with isolated synovitis of the third left metacarpophalangeal joint. Longitudinal bilocular constriction occurred along the extensor tendon proper. Distention by synovial saccules is seen on the ulnar and the radial side of the tendon.

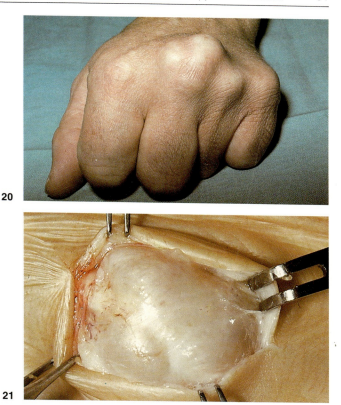

Fig. **20** Nodular articular synovitis of the third metacarpophalangeal joint. Here also a central longitudinal constriction by the extensor tendon occurred, with synovial saccules of varying sizes in a 43-year-old female.

Fig. **21** Operative finding at synovectomy. Extensor tendon pursuing a longitudinal course, displaced sideward. The lateral portions of the dorsal aponeurosis are maximally overstretched as the result of synovitis.

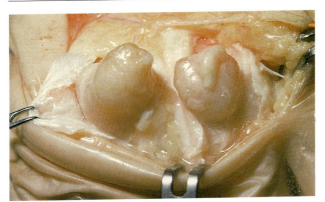

22

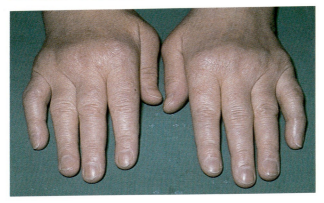

23

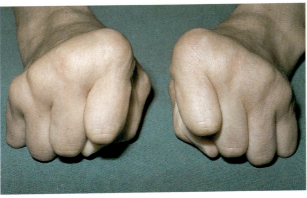

24

Proximal Interphalangeal Joint

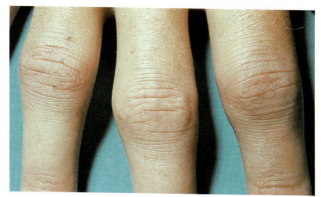

25

Fig. **22**   After the dorsal aponeurosis has been opened, the inflamed synovial tissue is forcibly extruded.

Fig. **23**   Symmetric involvement of the metacarpophalangeal joints by synovitis.

Fig. **24**   When a firm fist is made, the metacarpophalangeal joints, which are distended by synovitis, show a tendency to ulnar deviation.

Fig. **25**   Articular synovitis of the second to fourth interphalangeal joint with fusiform distention in a 24-year-old female.

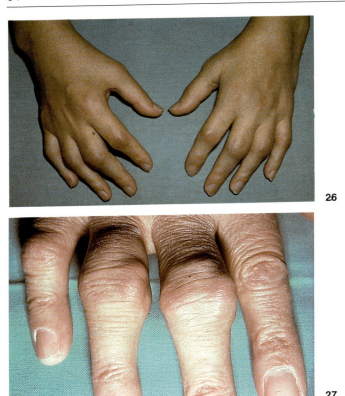

26

27

Fig. **26** Symmetric involvement of all proximal interphalangeal joints, which concomitantly show a dark discoloration, with fusiform distention. Incipient impairment of extension (the interphalangeal joints can no longer be fully extended).

Fig. **27** Nodular distention of the third and fourth proximal interphalangeal joint with herniation of the inflamed synovial tissue through the partially insufficient dorsal aponeurosis.

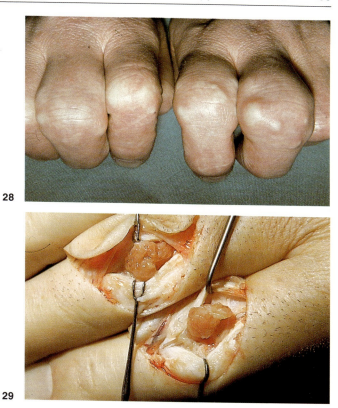

28

29

Fig. **28** On maximal flexion of the proximal interphalangeal joint, the multiple herniations are still better demonstrable (46-year-old female).

Fig. **29** After longitudinal incision of the insufficient area of the dorsal aponeurosis on the radial and the ulnar sides of the extensor tendon proper, the tissue that produces the synovial herniations becomes visible.

Distal Interphalangeal Joint

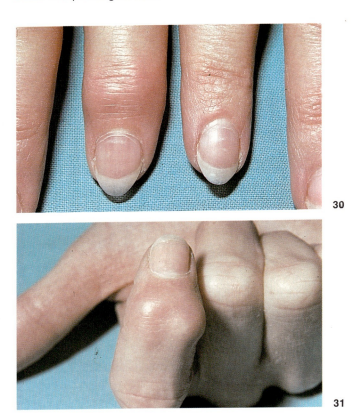

30

31

Fig. **30** Relatively infrequent involvement of the distal interphalangeal joint in seronegative rheumatoid arthritis. Second right distal interphalangeal joint is compared with the second left distal interphalangeal joint. Extreme distention and redness of the joint as well as of the surrounding soft tissues occurred as a consequence of the inflammatory reaction. The natural creasing of the skin is largely abolished. In the differential diagnosis the question arises whether this is a case of psoriatic arthritis without psoriasis or whether psoriasis of the skin will develop later.

Fig. **31** With maximal flexion, articular synovitis is distinctly manifested at both sides of the extensor tendon. (35-year-old female with rheumatoid arthritis).

Tenosynovitis and its Consequences

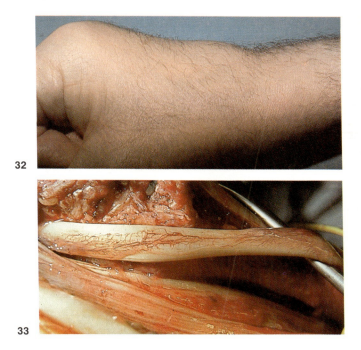

32

33

Fig. **32** Incipient tenosynovitis in a 64-year-old male with rheumatoid arthritis. The tenosynovial tissue has only proliferated distally to the transverse dorsal retinaculum in the region of the extensor tendons. The condition is less conspicuous in the superior or anterior views, but is seen distinctly on lateral inspection.

Fig. **33** Incidental finding in a 77-year-old female operated on for bilateral carpal tunnel syndrome. Joint complaints or swelling as an indication of rheumatoid arthritis so far had not occurred. During the operation, delicate vegetations of tenosynovitis with newly formed vessels, were encountered on the tendons in the carpal tunnel; these increased in thickness distally and proximally. It was therefore necessary to perform not only decompression and neurolysis of the median nerve, but also a total tenosynovectomy of the flexors. Subsequently, continued follow-up confirmed the presumptive diagnosis of rheumatoid arthritis that had been made on the basis of the operative findings.

Extensor Tendons

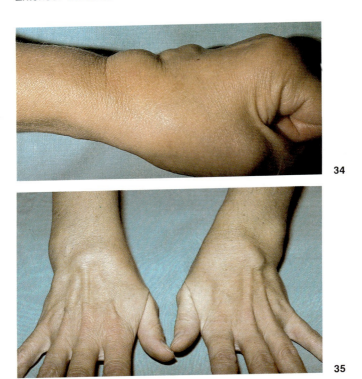

34

35

Fig. **34** 55-year-old female with rheumatoid arthritis. Loculated synovitis proximally and distally to the dorsal retinaculum, corresponding to involvement of
the extensor tendons.

Fig. **35** 36-year-old female with tenosynovitis of both wrist joints, prevalently
distally to the dorsal retinaculum. The cuff-shaped tendon sheath consisting of
two leaves has proliferated in circular fashion around the extensor tendons of
the individual long fingers. The latter are thus distinctly raised from the underlying tissues. On flexing and extending the fingers, parts of the tendon sheaths,
which are connected to individual or all tendons, take part in the movement.
Proximally to the retinaculum, a swelling due to tenosynovitis is barely recognizable. A conspicuous feature, particularly in the left hand, is the tenosynovitis-
induced distention in the surroundings of the tendon of the extensor carpi
ulnaris muscle.

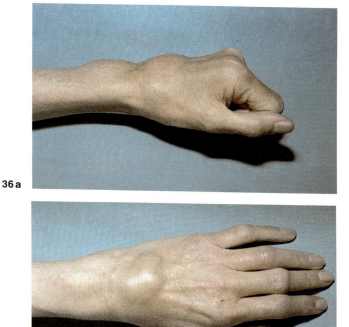

36 a

36 b

Figs. **36 a** and **b** 56-year-old female with rheumatoid arthritis. Bilocular constriction of the tenosynovitis-induced distention by the dorsal retinaculum. The
extensors of the long fingers and the thumb are involved.
The bilocular constriction is also visible in the dorsal view.

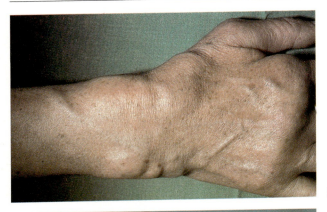

37

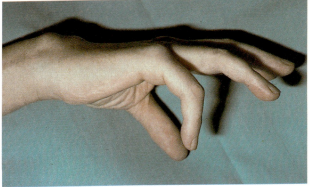

38

Fig. **37** 48-year-old female with rheumatoid arthritis. The tenosynovitis of the extensors is largely limited to the extensor aspect of the first ray and the tendon of the extensor carpi ulnaris muscle, whereas the extensor tendons of the four long fingers and the remaining extensors of the wrist present no major involvement.

Fig. **38** 56-year-old female with rheumatoid arthritis. Rupture of the extensor tendon of the fifth finger.

Fig. **39** Rupture of the extensors of the fourth and fifth fingers.

Fig. **40** Rupture of the extensors of three long fingers (III–V).

Fig. **41** Rupture of the extensor tendons of all long fingers (II–V). Dorsal dislocation of the head of the ulna (caput ulnae syndrome).

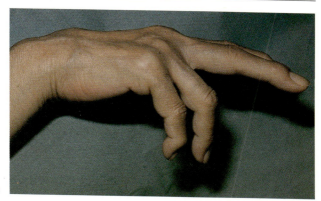

39

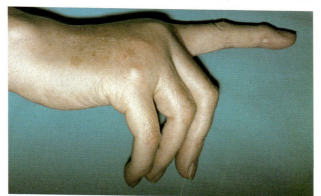

40

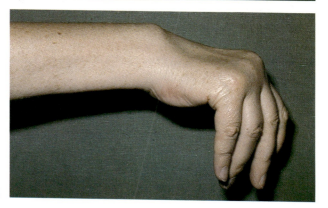

41

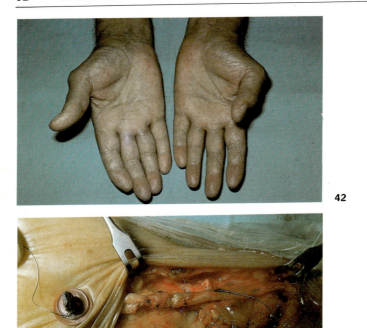

42

43

Fig. **42** Rupture of the tendon of the left extensor pollicis longus muscle. Maximum active extension of the left thumb is not possible. Even when the metacarpophalangeal joint is being fixed, the left distal phalanx can be flexed but not extended at the interphalangeal joint. Incipient subluxation at the metacarpophalangeal joint of the right thumb is the result of articular synovitis.

Flexor Tendons

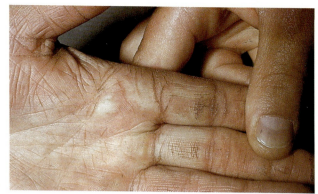

44

Fig. **43**   Timely tendon transfer, i.e., translocation of the tendons of a functioning muscle to the distal portion of the ruptured extensor tendons, can often, to a large extent or completely, compensate for the functional deficiency. In the present case, the tendon of the flexor carpi ulnaris muscle was transplanted to the ruptured extensor tendons of the third, fourth, and fifth fingers, with interlacing of the tendon after Pulvertaft and an extension suture after Lengemann. On the left is seen the plumb button on the skin, which holds the distal portion of the tendon in position, and on the right the proximal part of the extension suture that subsequently is carried through the skin, with the support seated on the tendon and individual adaptive sutures. Below is an intact tendon.

Fig. **44**   Occasionally, inflammatory nodular distentions of the sheath of the flexor tendons can only be made visible by maximal passive hyperextension of the fingers at the metacarpophalangeal joint. In the present case there is a tenosynovitis with the index finger locked in flexed position, due to rheumatoid arthritis in a 32-year-old female.

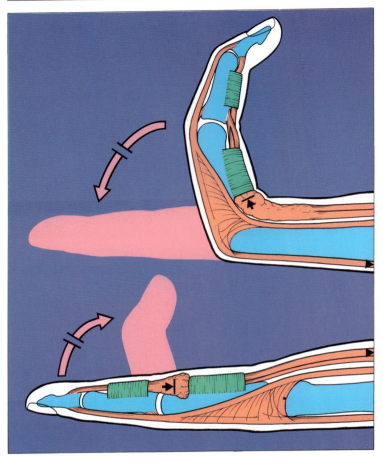

45

Fig. **45**   Tenosynovitis of the flexors of the fingers. Consequence: the trigger finger syndrome. Top: blocking in the extended position. Flexion not possible. Bottom: blocking in the flexed position. Extension not possible. The inflamed tenosynovial tissue cannot glide through the fibrous tendon sheath.

Figs. **46a** and **b**   Marked tenosynovitis of both flexor tendons of the third digit. The swelling results from fluid being held back by the annular ligaments in the distal palm and becomes distinctly prominent on the volar side of the proximal phalanx.

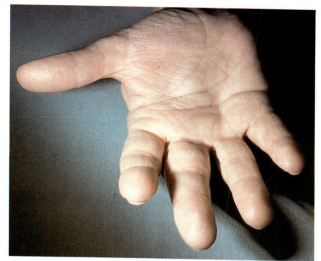

46 a

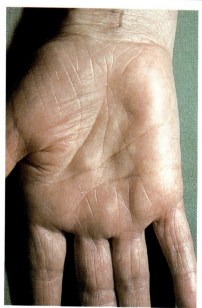

46 b

Figs. **47a** and **b**   Savill's test.
a) In the presence of a tenosynovitis, no skin fold can be raised on lateral compression of the soft tissues on the flexor aspect of the finger by the examiner's thumb and index finger.
b) A skin fold can be raised in the index finger. This cannot be done in the third finger because of distention from tenosynovitis.

Fig. **48**   Isolated tenosynovitis of the flexor tendons of a digit in the proximal region (palm) or the distal region (finger) is an infrequent event. Masses of inflamed tenosynovial tissue can be removed at operation.

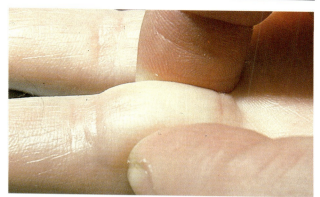

47a

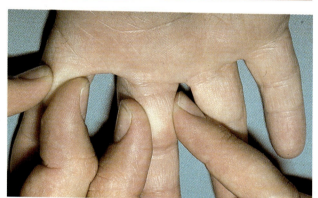

47b

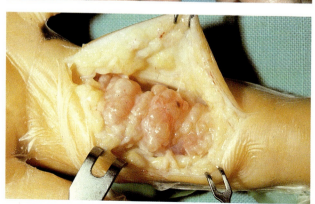

48

Fig. **49**   Besides the necessary tenosynovectomy of both tendons, including the glide way between the tendons and bones or joints, the annular ligaments, excepting a small rest, have often to be resected. When the deep ligaments are involved in addition, it is essential that their point of penetration through the split of the superficial tendon be cleaned of inflamed tenosynovial tissue. In the postoperative period, these conditions require a complex individualized treatment with remedial exercises because adhesion of the postsynovectomy wounds of both tendons can, if at all, only be treated in this manner. The successful result of surgical treatment, especially in the region of the flexor tendons, cannot be predicted, since it also depends on the activity and the selective exercises on the part of the patient.

Patients with a tenosynovitis often are brought to operation relatively late. There already exists extreme invasive growth of inflamed tenosynovial tissue into the individual tendons, accompanied by extensive destruction. The latter is, however, not recognizable by functional impairment. At this moment, the infiltration of the tendon structure with inflamed synovial tissue still compensates for the decreased stability of this structure. Tenosynovectomy aims at radical removal of the entire inflamed synovial tissue. It is understandable that this procedure impairs the structure of the tendon and its stability. Nevertheless, tenosynovectomy is the only means of arresting the otherwise inevitable destruction. After tenosynovectomy, it is not always possible to avoid further damage to the tendons by overstretching. This makes the exceptional postoperative rupture of a previously damaged tendon understandable.

Fig. **50**   Postoperative condition following W-shaped incision for isolated tenosynovitis of the flexors of the third digit.

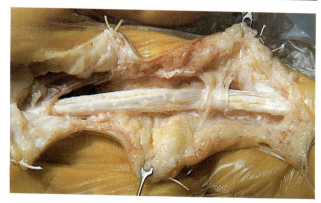

49

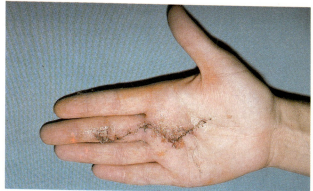

50

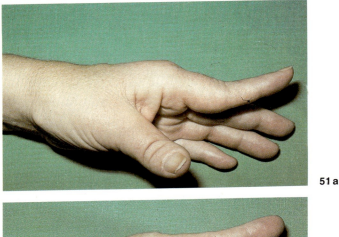

51a

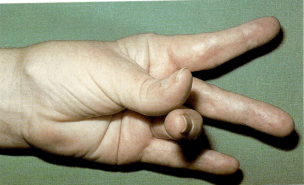

51b

Figs. **51a** and **b** 51-year-old female with rheumatoid arthritis. Loss of function of most flexor tendons. Extreme malposition with hyperextension of the index finger. Rupture of the deep and the superficial flexor tendons of the first, second, third, and fifth fingers. Only the superficial flexor tendon of the fourth finger has been spared. When the patient is asked to make a firm fist, only the fourth finger and the thumb are moved (the latter by the muscles of the thenar eminence). Whereas the functional deficiency resulting from rupture of individual or several extensor tendons can be largely compensated for by early surgery and exercise therapy, this favorable result is not always to be expected in rupture of the flexor tendons. Primary tendon suture is impractical so that at times one must aim at achieving a favorable result by a two-stage operation. However, despite all precautions, postoperative adhesion of one or both tendons to each other or their surroundings cannot always be prevented.

Other Changes of the Hand

Ulnar Deviation

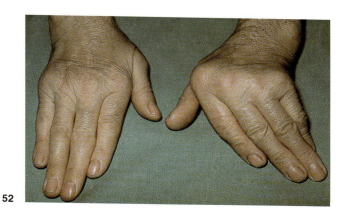

52

Fig. **52**   Marked ulnar deviation of the long fingers of the left hand with distinct impairment of extension at the metacarpophalangeal joints.

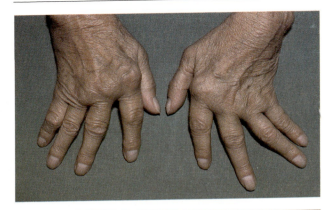

53 a

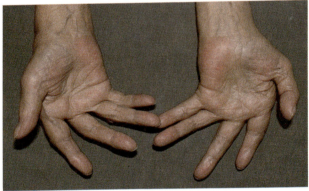

53 b

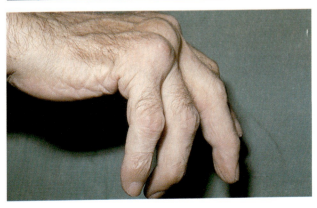

54

Buttonhole Deformity

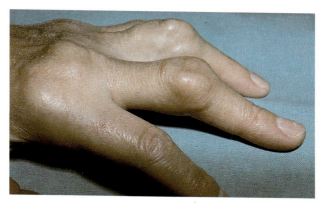

55

Figs. **53a** and **b**   Articular synovitis of the metacarpophalangeal joints with ulnar deviation of the long fingers. **a)** The patient corrects the anomaly more or less unconsciously by placing her hands on a surface. **b)** On placing the backs of the hands on a surface, the full extent of the incorrectable ulnar deviation is manifested.

Fig. **54**   Extremely deficient extension of the long fingers as the result of ulnar deviation with slipping of the extensor tendons into the ulnar interdigital spaces. The deficient extension developing in this manner must not be confused with the similar deficiency in rupture of the second to fifth extensor tendons.

Fig. **55**   Deficient extension of the proximal and middle phalanges as the result of synovitis of the metacarpophalangeal and proximal interphalangeal joints. Distinct insufficiency of the dorsal aponeurosis paving the way for a buttonhole deformity.

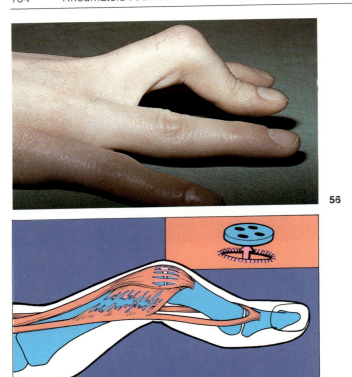

56

57

Fig. **56**   Marked buttonhole deformity of the fourth finger:
– hyperextension at the metacarpophalangeal joint,
– flexion at the proximal interphalangeal joint,
– hyperextension at the distal interphalangeal joint of the finger involved.

Fig. **57**   The insufficiency of the dorsal aponeurosis gives rise to lateral deviation of the radial as well as the ulnar ligaments and the dorsal aponeurosis comes to lie below the axis of the proximal interphalangeal joint. These ligaments pull the middle phalanx into a position of flexion and the proximal as well as the distal phalanx into a position of hyperextension so that the latter phalanx perforates the dorsal aponeurosis like a button through a buttonhole (buttonhole deformity).

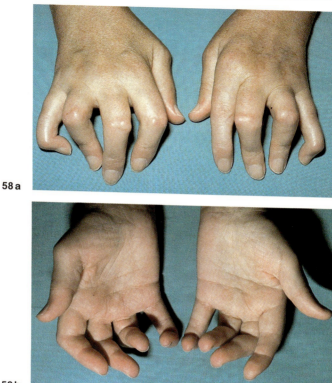

58 a

58 b

Figs. **58 a** and **b**   Largely symmetrically arranged, fixed buttonhole deformity present in nearly all the proximal interphalangeal joints of both hands without a possibility for passive compensation. Concomitant rupture of the extensor tendons in the regions of the distal interphalangeal joints of both fifth fingers.
a) The condyles of the heads of the proximal phalanges are visible through the skin over the dorsal sides of the proximal interphalangeal joints.
b) Opening of both hands is considerably restricted. This is a 46-year-old female with rheumatoid arthritis.

Swan-Neck Deformity

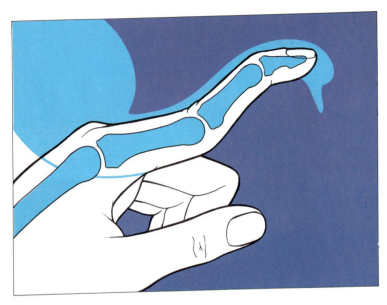

59

Fig. **59**   The swan-neck deformity is characterized by:
— flexion at the metacarpophalangeal joint,
— hyperextension at the proximal interphalangeal joint,
— flexion at the distal interphalangeal joint
of the finger involved. In the beginning, the faulty position can be corrected
passively. In an advanced stage the patient is incapable of making a fist so that
the function of the hand is considerably impaired.

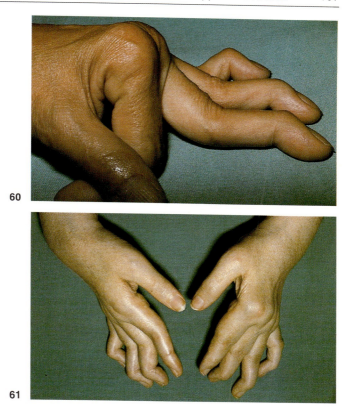

Fig. 60 Swan-neck deformity partially correctable by passive motion in a 58-year-old female.

Fig. 61 45-year-old female with a swan-neck deformity of all long fingers, which is no longer passively correctable. The swan-neck deformity is due, among other factors, to contracture of the intrinsic musculature (interosseous and lumbrical muscles).

Double-Rectangled Deformity

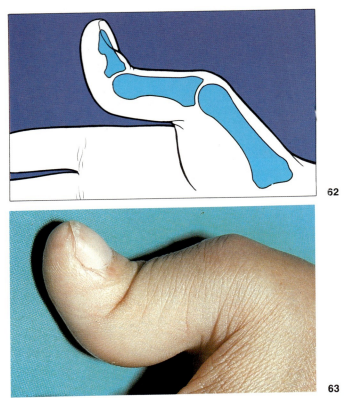

Fig. **62** The double rectangled deformity of the thumb is also typical of the rheumatoid hand.
It consists in:
− a flexed position at the metacarpophalangeal joint, and
− a hyperextended position at the interphalangeal joint,
both malpositions of approximately 90°. When the malposition is no longer actively correctable, primarily because of the instability of both joints of the thumb but also because of supervening deformations, the result is considerable restriction of the function of the thumb and thereby of the entire hand. Prehension of an object with use of the index finger and the flexor aspect of the interphalangeal joint of the thumb (provided the index finger is not involved). The key grip is also considerably impaired.

Fig. **63** Double right-angled deformity of the left thumb viewed dorsally.

Combined and Extreme Lesions in the Region of the Hand

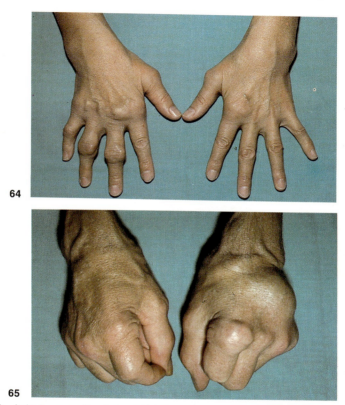

64

65

Fig. **64**   Articular synovitis of several joints but with partly asymmetric involvement. The metacarpophalangeal joints I–IV and the proximal interphalangeal joints II–V of the right hand are affected. Deficient extension of the third to fifth finger at the proximal interphalangeal joints of the right hand are the result of synovitis.

Fig. **65**   48-year-old female with rheumatoid arthritis with involvement of both hands. In the left hand there is marked loculated tenosynovitis of the extensors, constricted by the oblique course of the dorsal retinaculum. Articular synovitis of the metacarpophalangeal joints I–IV. In the right hand there is articular synovitis of the metacarpophalangeal joints I–III and the proximal interphalangeal joint of the index finger. Incipient formation of rheumatoid nodules on the prehensile surface of the distal phalanx of the thumb and discrete tenosynovitis of the extensors over the wrist joint are present.

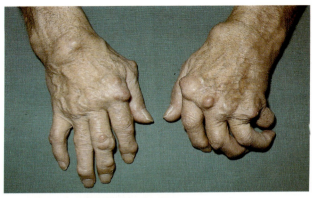

66

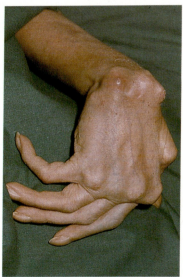

Fig. **66** A 56-year-old male with seropositive rheumatoid arthritis has tenosynovitis and articular synovitis in both wrist joints. The radial side of the right hand and the ulnar side of the left hand are predominantly affected. Dislocation of the metacarpophalangeal joints II–V with ulnar deviation of the fingers has developed on the basis of past synovitis of all metacarpophalangeal joints and some of the proximal interphalangeal joints. Replacement of the metacarpophalangeal joints II–V of the right hand by Swanson prostheses has produced a favorable result. The appearance of multiple rheumatoid nodules over the extensor surfaces of the wrist and individual finger joints is an unusual event.

67

Fig. **67** 46-year-old male with rheumatoid arthritis and bayonet displacement at the wrist due to increased deformity of the distal ulna and dislocation with unusually strong ulnar deviation of the wrist. The view of the distal articular surfaces of radius and ulna shows rheumatoid nodules over the ulnar articular surface. The metacarpophalangeal joints of the long fingers are also extremely dislocated toward the ulna. Extension at the wrist and at some of the metacarpophalangeal joints is not possible. The hand is of hardly any use without operative intervention.

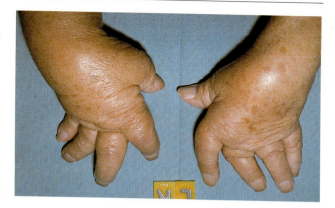

68 a

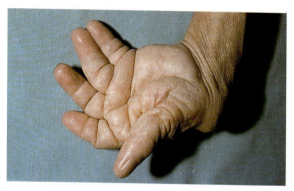

68 b

Figs. **68 a** and **b** 69-year-old female with disabling rheumatoid arthritis. There exists extreme deformation with a tendency of both hands to shrinking. The wrist joint, the carpal bones, and some of the metacarpophalangeal joints, including their capsuloligamental apparatus, are destroyed so that the joints have become completely unstable. The entire function of the hand is thus impaired. Larger objects can only be grasped with considerable effort, and subtle prehensile movements can no longer be performed.

Fortunately, the last-named extreme lesions are of relatively rare occurrence. Not every case of rheumatoid arthritis results in these deformations. In other cases such extreme alterations do not develop because therapeutic procedures, especially operations, prevent a major deterioration of shape and function.

Articular Synovitis, Tenosynovitis, and their Sequelae in the Lower Extremities

Hip Joint

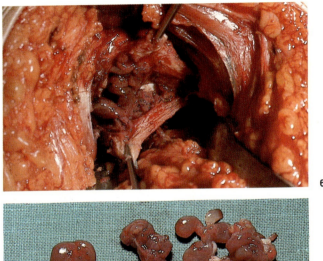

69

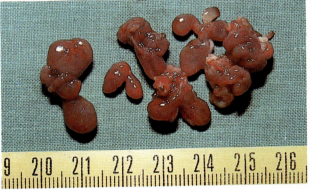

70

Fig. **69** Marked synovitis with formation of distinct villi after opening of the fibrotic contracted capsule of the hip joint.

Fig. **70** Specimen of villi obtained at synovectomy of the hip joint.

Figs. **71a** and **b** Complete loss of roundness of the femoral head as the result of coxitis in a 30-year-old female with rheumatoid arthritis. Destruction with depression of the cranial parts of the femoral head, is shown. Especially in the presence of bilateral alterations, only total hip arthroplasty – to be sure, an absolute contraindication in younger individuals – can bring about an improvement of mobility, which otherwise is definitely lost.

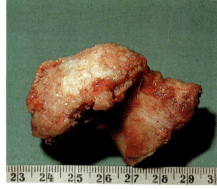

71a

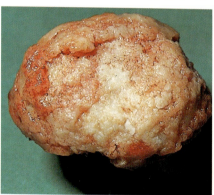

71b

Fig. **72** Destruction and considerable decrease in size of the femoral head in a 38-year-old female with rheumatoid arthritis. Marked synovitis with marginal erosions is seen. The articular surface is no longer covered with cartilage but has undergone eburnation.

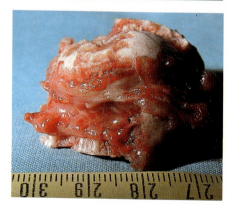

72

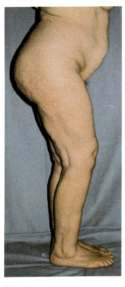

73

Fig. **73**   Flexion contracture of both hip joints as the result of synovitis, accompanied by destructive and degenerative lesions. Incipient reactive flexed position of the knee joints and hyperlordosis with deficient erection of the trunk are shown.

Figs. **74 a–c**   Adduction contracture of the right hip joint in coxitis as the result of rheumatoid arthritis. Left-sided obliquity of the pelvis (which can also be recognized by the course of the rima ani) and resultant relative lengthening of the left leg. Leg lengthening and synovitis lead to flexion contracture and varus position of the left knee joint. The relative shortening of the right leg can be recognized by the compensatory raising of the heel of the foot.

Figs. **75 a** and **b**   Distinct flexion contracture with advanced adduction contracture of the left hip joint as the result of rheumatoid coxitis in a 51-year-old female. Adduction contracture and pelvic obliquity have led to relative lengthening of the right leg. This lengthening, together with the concomitant coxitis and gonarthritis, has produced a marked flexion contracture of both joints and a malposition of the right hip joint in external rotation, which masks the valgus deformity of both knees.

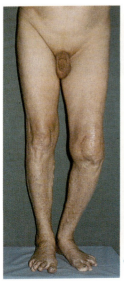

74a

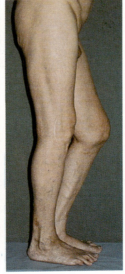

74b

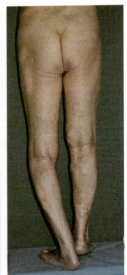

74c

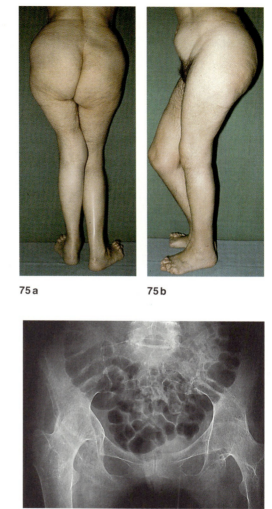

75a   75b

76

Fig. **76** Rheumatoid arthritis with bony ankylosis of both hip joints. Concomitant extreme osteoporosis as the consequence of disease and immobilization.

Knee Joint

Synovitis

Fig. **77**   45-year-old female with incipient rheumatoid arthritis with diffuse swelling of the right knee joint, including its surroundings. The contours are obliterated.

Figs. **78**   53-year-old male with rheumatoid arthritis. Marked swelling of the left knee joint, is chiefly limited to the medial part of the upper recess.

Fig. **79**   46-year-old female with rheumatoid arthritis. The level of the patella is lower than the swelling. The maximal swelling has already led to decreased extensibility and an incipient position on flexion.

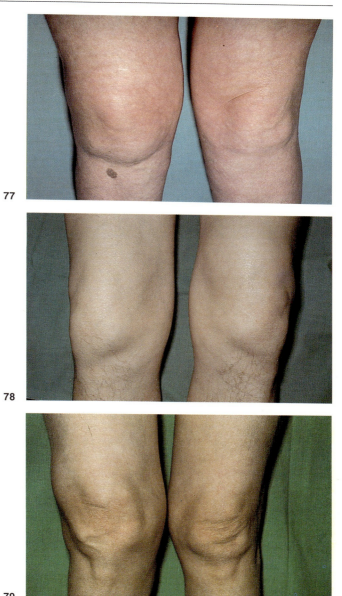

77

78

79

Arthrocele (Baker's cyst)

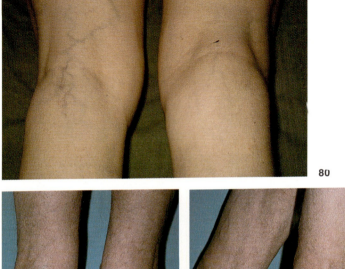

80

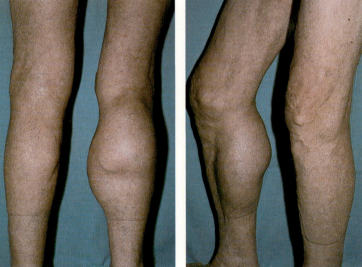

81 a

81

Fig. **80**   Pouching of the capsule of the knee joint in the right popliteal space with extensive Baker's cyst. The diagnosis can be confirmed by a lateral roentgenogram of the knee joint and by arthrography, sonography, and operation.

Figs. **81 a** and **b**   Baker's cyst expanding as far as the medial and also the distal part of the calf. Examination raises the strong suspicion of loculation.

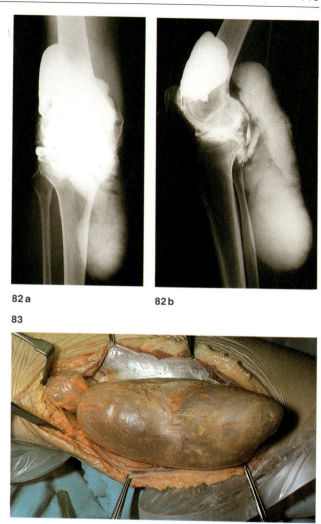

82 a   **82 b**

83

Figs. **82 a** and **b** Arthrography demonstrates the expansion of the upper recess and of Baker's cyst.

Fig. **83** Dissection of the cyst in the regions of the popliteal space and the calf. An additional pouching is visible in the popliteal space.

Fig. **84**   Deep dissection confirms the clinical suspicion of loculation.

Fig. **85**   Loculated cysts containing masses of fibrin and joint fluid.

Fig. **86**   The capsule is relatively thin. Gross inspection reveals no synovitis in the wall, but histologically the lining of the cyst is comparable to the synovial lining of the joint (Mohr). These cysts usually contain only fibrin and fluid, whereas inflamed synovial tissue does line the cyst wall but does not constitute a major part in the contents of the cyst.

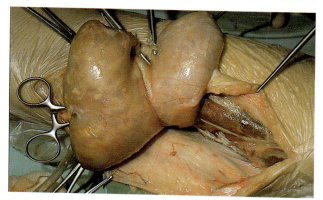

84

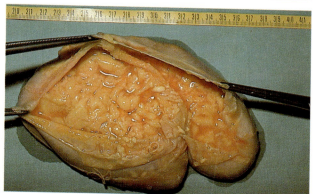

85

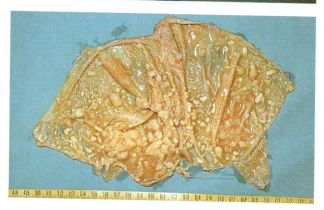

86

Faulty Positions

Fig. **87**   This female with rheumatoid arthritis already presents a bilateral genu valgum when the legs are weighted. Conspicuous pigmentation of both lower legs containing iron (verified histologically).

Fig. **88**   Increasing destruction of both knee joints with bilateral valgus position gives rise to a relative increase of the distance between the internal malleoli when the knees are approximated. There is marked atrophy of the muscles in the upper leg. A bilateral total hip arthroplasty can enable the patient to walk again.

Figs. **89a** and **b**   41-year-old female with rheumatoid arthritis. Extreme varus position of the right leg.

Figs. **90a** and **b**   Flexion contracture of the knee joints, especially when combined with a varus or valgus position, can give rise to changes in the neighboring joints. The disorder in both knee joints in a 64-year-old female produced a reactive flexion contracture of the hip joints that were not involved in the inflammation. To prevent reactive secondary damages, exercise treatment should be instituted at an early stage. When the impairment proves irreversible, the faulty position should be corrected surgically. However, total arthroplasty is avoided, if possible.

87

88

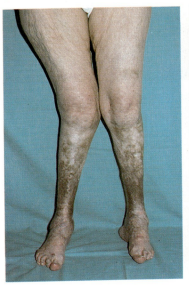
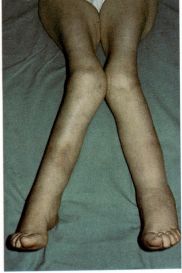

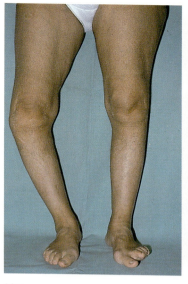
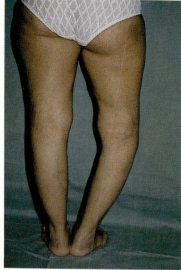

89 a **89 b**
90 a **90 b**

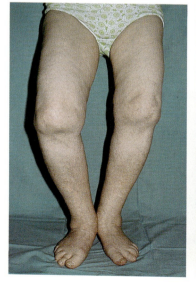
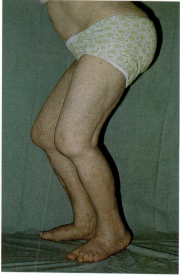

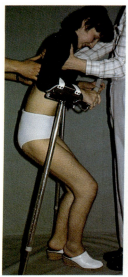 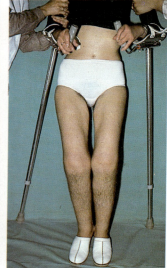

91 a   **91 b**

92

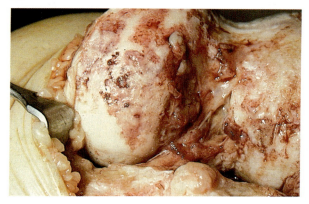

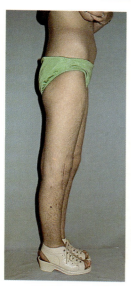

93 a

93 b

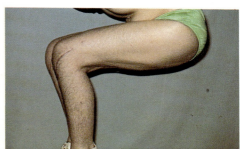

Figs. **91 a** and **b**   Unfortunately, with increasing frequency we see younger individuals with extreme deformations that impede their mobilization, so that total arthroplasty cannot always be avoided, although the indication for this procedure has to be quite exceptional. A 27-year-old female with rheumatoid arthritis was immobilized on the advice of several nonmedical practitioners and a physician because of a flexion contracture of both knee joints and a secondary malposition of the hip joints in the presence of high inflammatory activity. Exercise therapy was discouraged. This method of treatment is not justifiable despite the possible occurrence of intense pain. Before long the immobilization produced considerable atrophy of the entire musculature of the upper leg, and especially the quadriceps muscle. The patient can only stay on her feet with difficulty, using an ambulation aid and assisted by two persons.

Fig. **92**   Despite the contractures and the major destruction of the articular surfaces by the progressive synovitis encountered at arthrotomy (the destruction of the cartilage being nearly complete), implantation of artificial knee joints was omitted and synovectomy with arthrolysis was performed on both knee joints instead. These two-stage operations were only undertaken after the muscular function had improved. The patient (Fig. **93**) became capable of walking again.

Figs. **93 a** and **b**   For more than 2 years the patient has now been capable of walking a considerable distance and can even drive a car a long way. Ambulation was additionally improved by bilateral resection of the metatarsal heads because of a rheumatoid deformity of the forefoot, and by synovectomy of an ankle joint, both in one stage.

Ankle Joint

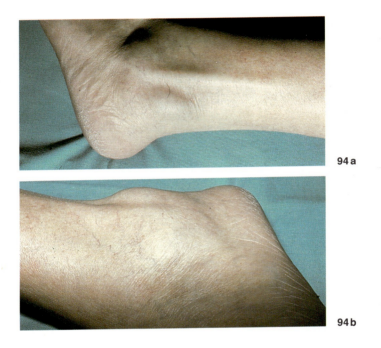

94 a

94 b

Figs. **94 a** and **b**   Distinct swelling behind the left lateral malleolus from tenc-synovitis of the fibular extensor tendons in a 65-year-old female with rheumatoid arthritis. Crepitation can often be felt when the hand is placed on the swelling and the foot is moved concomitantly.

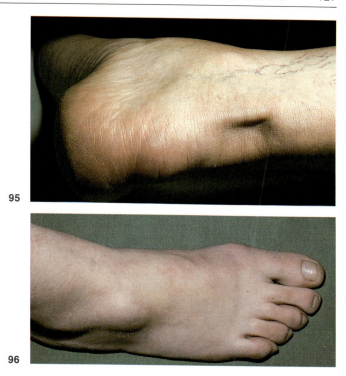

95

96

Fig. **95** 47-year-old female with rupture of the Achilles tendon due to rheumatiod arthritis. Break of the contour is in the form of a depression in which the proximal and the distal stump of the tendon are recognizable. Distally, there is a projection formed by the retracting stump. Above the depression, one notes the preserved tendon of the plantaris muscle. Owing to the rupture, plantar flexion against resistance is not possible, particularly when the patient attempts to stand on her toes.

Fig. **96** 41-year-old female with a circumscribed swelling in the anterolateral portion of the tibiotalar joint. The rheumatoid arthritis has given rise to synovitis of the tendon and the joint in this region.

Fig. **97** Articular synovitis as well as tenosynovitis in the region of the talo-crural joint can be treated by synovectomy. When needed, we prefer four incisions, two anterior to and two posterior to the medial and the lateral malleolus. The operation is performed on both feet simultaneously by two teams. In view of the multiplicity of operations required for arthritic patients, tne number of general anesthesias can thus be reduced and the period of hospita'i-zation becomes appreciably shortened. In the present case, the operation was also performed simultaneously on both feet, using four incisions (mattress type of continuous wire suture, sixth postoperative day).

Fig. **98** 65-year-old female with incipient varus position of the left tibiotalar joint during the degenerative phase of rheumatoid arthritis.

Fig. **99** 54-year-old female with advanced rheumatoid arthritis displaying extreme valgus of the tibiotalar joint, accompanied by increasing instability that permits standing and walking only with considerable discomfort. At the moment, there is no marked synovitis of the tibiotalar joint.

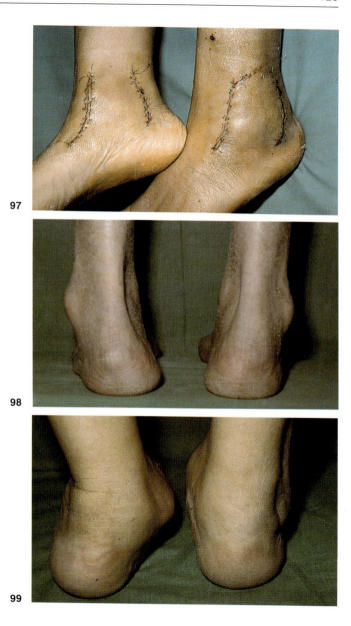

97

98

99

Figs. **100a** and **b**   Rheumatoid flatfoot resulting from instability of the entire capsuloligamental apparatus of the weight-bearing foot in a 66-year-old female with rheumatoid arthritis. The plantar arches of both feet are completely demolished. In addition, the foot tilts lateralward, so that the internal malleolus, the talus, and the navicular bone project distinctly on the medial border of the foot. Bursae are formed in the vicinity of the navicular bone.

Fig. **101**   View of the plantar side in marked valgus position of both ankle joints with bulging of the internal malleoli and formation of bursae over the projecting tarsal bones at the medial border of the foot, which are becoming detached from their connections.

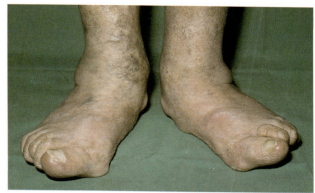

100a

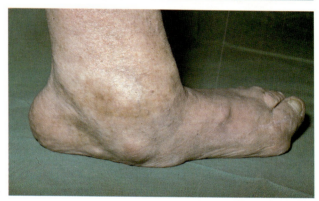

100b

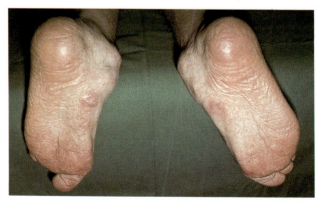

101

Region of the Forefoot

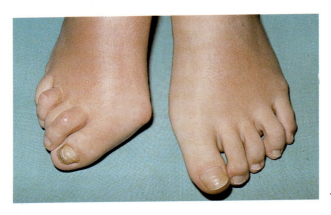

102

Fig. **102**   Development of a so-called rheumatoid forefoot on the right side with fibular deviation of all toes as a sequel of rheumatoid arthritis in a young female. In addition, extreme hallux valgus with formation of a bursa over the first metacarpophalangeal joint and a hammer toe deformity of the second and fourth toes with clavus formation. There are no major changes on the contralateral side. The entire right foot is slightly swollen and reddened. Normal and painless weight bearing is no longer possible.

Fig. **103**   Predominant involvement of the right foot with extreme hallux valgus and rotation of the great toe. Projecting bursae are on the medial side of the first metatarsophalangeal joint. Digitus superductus of the second and third toes over the hallux. Slight medial deviation and dislocation of the four small toes. Hammer toe deformity of the second and third toe with corns over the proximal interphalangeal joints. As the result of their dorsal dislocation, the four small toes are located as it were "on the second floor" over the metatarsal heads, which are dislocated plantarward. The right forefoot is distinctly broadened in comparison with the left forefoot.

Fig. **104**   Symmetric alterations of both forefeet: tibial deviation and dorsal dislocation of the eight small toes, hallux valgus and digitus superductus, incipient ulcerations over the prominent areas of the forefeet, which are exposed to strain and covered with bursae. Marked bony prominence with reactive formation of a bursa in the region of both second tarsometatarsal joints on the dorsum of the feet.

Fig. **105**   Fibular deviation of all toes with malrotation of the big toes in addition to bilateral hallux valgus. An ulcer that refuses to heal has been present for several months in the medial region of the first left metatarsophalangeal joint. In the left foot, there is digitus superductus position of the second and third toes upon the fourth and fifth toes.

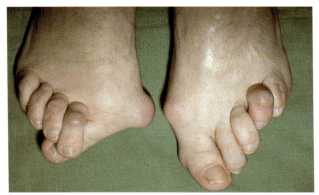

103

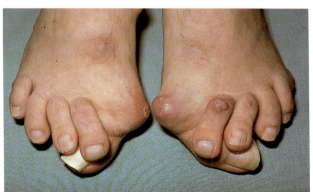

104

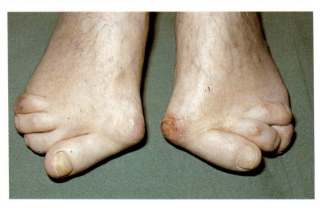

105

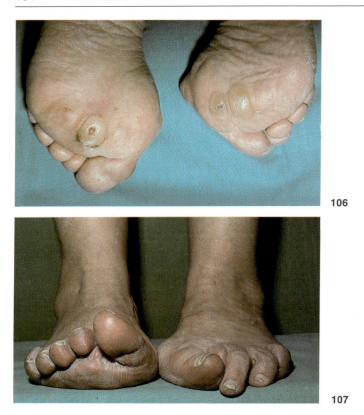

106

107

Fig. **106** Improper pedicure frequently gives rise to refractory skin lesions over the plantarward dislocated heads of the metatarsals, which refuse to heal and can lead to protracted disorders of wound healing with infection.

Fig. **107** The frontal view shows the dorsal dislocation of the small toes (located superiorly) with respect to the heads of the metatarsals.

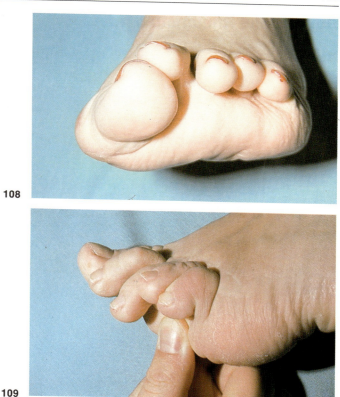

108

109

Fig. **108**   Pressure exerted from the distal region of the sole upon the metatarsal heads effects partial correction of the dislocation, provided they have not yet become fixed by contracture.

Fig. **109**   The dorsal dislocation of the toes of the right foot prevents them from touching the ground during standing and walking. Therefore they cannot support heal-toe ambulation. In addition, the latter is impaired by the plantar dislocation of the metatarsal heads and by the reactive formation of bursae and callosities. With bilateral involvement the gait becomes awkward and stamping.

Bursitis and Rheumatoid Nodules

Bursitis

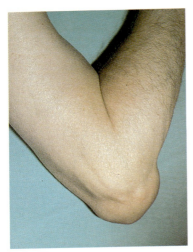

110

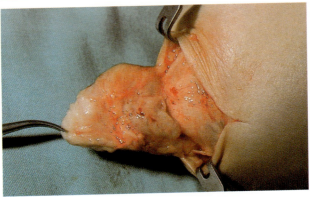

111

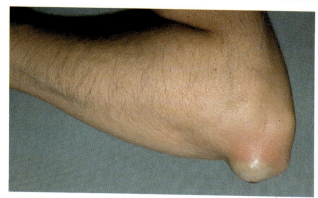

112

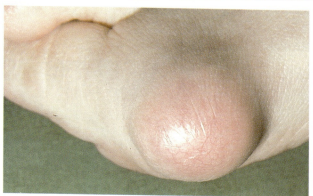

113

fig. **110** Development of bursae on the extensor aspect of the elbow joint in rheumatoid arthritis.

Fig. **111** When the bursa becomes annoying and painful by its increasing size, it can be extirpated.

Fig. **112** Olecranon bursitis shortly before perforation. The yellowish or reddish discoloration is not due to infection but solely to distention. Extirpation revealed a communication with the elbow joint. The effusion produced by the articular synovitis passed from the joint into the bursa, so that the latter was constantly filled to the maximum.

Fig. **113** Bursitis over the medial side of the first metatarsophalangeal joint in hallux valgus. In the latter deformity of the great toe, this region is exposed to maximum pressure.

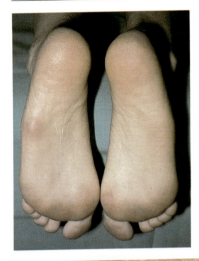

114

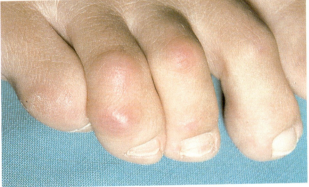

115

Fig. **114**   Development of a bursa on the plantar side of the left foot over the tuberosity of the fifth metatarsal.

Fig. **115**   Development of a bursa over the extensor sides of the third and fourth proximal interphalangeal joint and the fourth distal interphalangeal joint of the right foot in incipient rheumatoid arthritis.

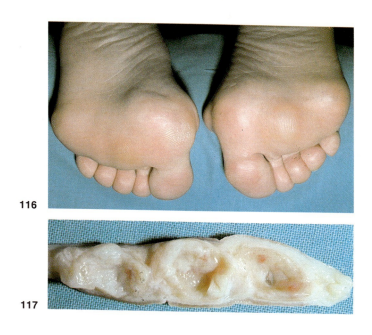

116

117

Fig. **116** Multiple inflamed bursae on the plantar side of both feet in active rheumatoid arthritis with concomitant marked synovitis of the metatarsophalangeal joints of the toes. The hypertrophic synovitis and the bursitis give rise to considerable discomfort on weight bearing.

Fig. **117** Four bursae are firmly adherent to the skin excised from the sole during resection of the metatarsal heads.

Rheumatoid Nodules

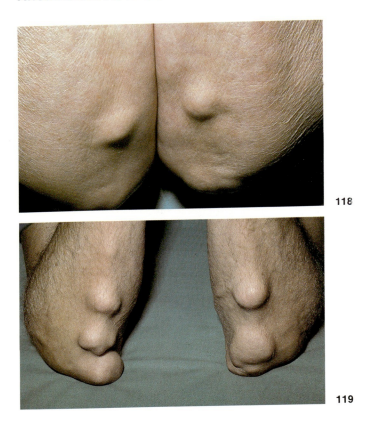

118

119

Fig. **118** Solitary rheumatoid nodules on the extensor surface in the proximal region of both forearms.

Fig. **119** Multiple rheumatoid nodules over the extensor surfaces of the elbow joints and the proximal forearms.

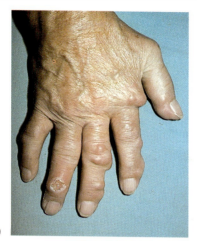

120

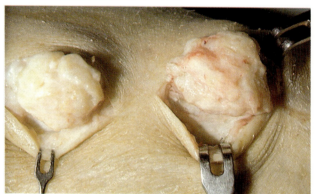

121

Fig. **120** Solitary, and particularly multiple, rheumatoid nodules occur much less frequently in the hand of the patient with rheumatoid arthritis. After an injury, an ulcer developed in a rheumatoid nodule over the distal interphalangeal joint of the fourth finger.

Fig. **121** Operative removal of two rheumatoid nodules over the extensor surfaces of two metacarpophalangeal joints.

Combinations

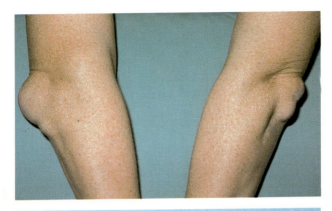

122

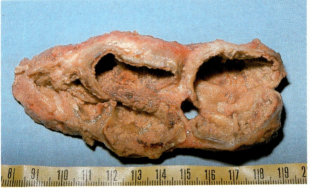

123

Fig. **122** Marked bursitis over both elbow joints. In their distal parts rheumatoid nodules are recognizable.

Fig. **123** Specimen of a loculated bursitis, the lining of which is disintegrating. Its wall contains rheumatoid nodules.

Juvenile Rheumatoid Arthritis

Juvenile rheumatoid arthritis (starting by the age of 16 years) occurs in different patterns, which vary considerably from adult rheumatoid arthritis. An arthritis limited chiefly to the joints has to be separated from a systemic clinical picture involving internal organs, which can scarcely be influenced by therapeutic measures.

Articular Synovitis and its Consequences

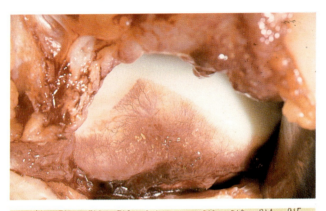

124

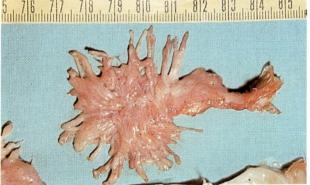

125

Fig. **124** Proliferative phase of synovitis of the knee joint in juvenile rheumatoid arthritis.

Fig. **125** Multiple villous proliferations of the synovial tissue in juvenile rheumatoid arthritis.

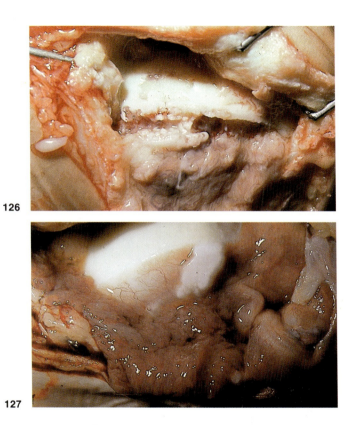

126

127

Fig. **126**   Marginal erosions and planar destruction of cartilage in the knee joint during the destructive phase.

Fig. **127**   Chondrophytic excrescences at the border between cartilage and bone with a filmy pannus of inflamed synovial tissue in the surroundings, the result of a new inflammatory episode during the degenerative phase.

Synovitis-Induced Clinical Changes

Changes Due to Tenosynovitis and Articular Synovitis

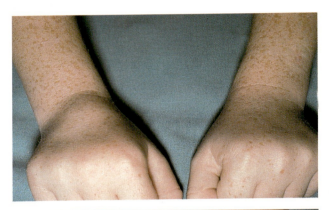

128

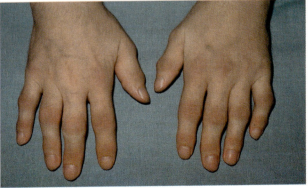

129

Fig. **128**   Typical swelling of inflamed tenosynovial tissue on the dorsal side of the right wrist in a 9-year-old girl.

Fig. **129**   Symmetric articular synovitis of the proximal interphalangeal joints and, to a lesser degree, of the distal interphalangeal joints, which are conspicuous by their dark discoloration.

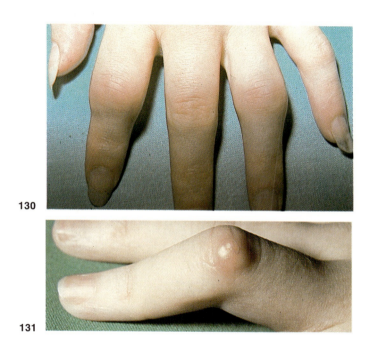

130

131

Fig. **130** Synovitis of the second and fourth proximal interphalangeal joints with incipient impairment of extension.

Fig. **131** Buttonhole deformity of the fourth finger in a 17-year-old girl with herniating synovitis.

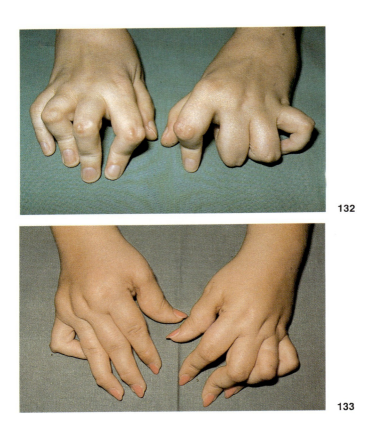

132

133

Fig. **132** Fixed buttonhole deformity of all long fingers. The condyles of the heads of the proximal phalanges have perforated the insufficient dcrsal aponeurosis.

Fig. **133** Buttonhole and swan-neck deformities in both hands.

Synovitis of the Knee Joint

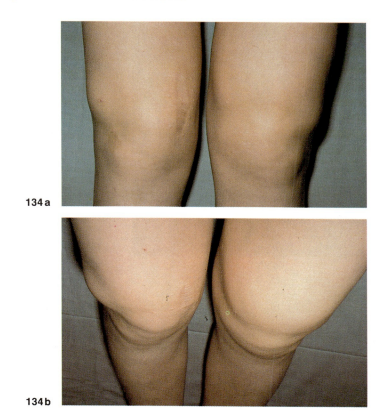

134 a

134 b

Figs. **134 a** and **b**   Marked synovitis of both knee joints. Swelling predominantly of the upper recess. Scar of exploratory arthrotomy of the right knee joint.

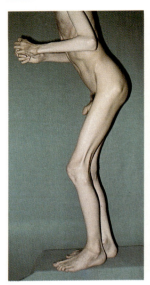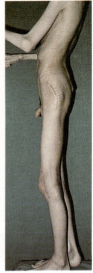

135 a + b

Figs. **135 a** and **b**   Bilateral flexion contracture of the hip and knee joints in a 17-year-old adolescent with juvenile rheumatoid arthritis.
a) Immediately prior to surgical treatment.
b) Ten weeks after the operation. The treatment consisted of synovectomy and arthrolysis of both hip joints and knee joints, the operation being performed on the hip and the knee of one extremity at the same time. Erect posture and gait are possible without an ambulation aid. The patient, who previously was hardly capable of walking, has been graduated from high school and has got his driver's license. He cares for himself during his study. Ankylosis of both elbow joints is present.

Fig. **136**   Influence of juvenile rheumatoid arthritis on growth. Posterior curvature of the proximal lower leg with shortening in a 19-year-old male. In addition, extension at the knee joint is considerably limited.

Fig. **137**   Equalization of leg length by placing blocks under the heel.

Fig. **138**   Hyperlordosis of the spine in flexion and adduction contracture of the hip joints, valgus of the knees, and flexion contracture of the elbow joints in a 24-year-old female with sequelae of juvenile rheumatoid arthritis.

Growth-Related Changes

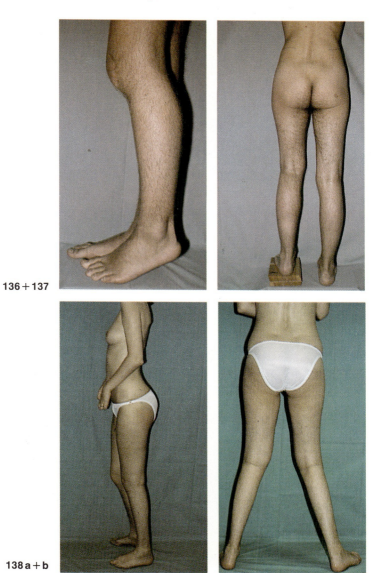

136 + 137

138 a + b

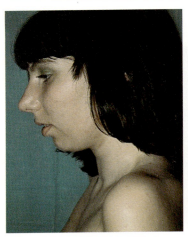

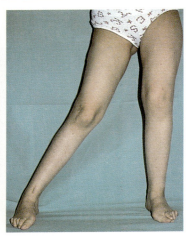

139

140

Fig. **139**   Micrognathia in the patient shown in Figure **138.**

Fig. **140**   Abducted position of the right hip joint with low level of the pelvis and considerable right-sided pes varus in a 13-year-old girl.

141

142

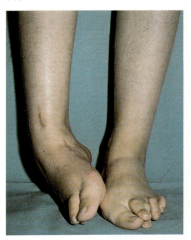

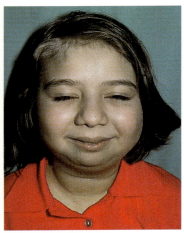

Ankylosing Juvenile Rheumatoid Arthritis

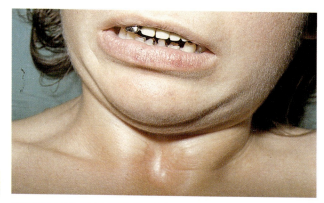

143

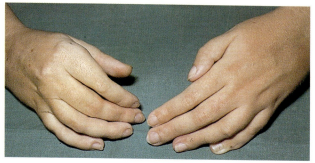

144

◀ Fig. **141** When the adducted malposition is equalized by obliquity of the pelvis, weight is borne by the lateral border of the foot. Displacement osteotomies on the hip and the foot, in the present case combined with tendon transfers, resulted in correction of the malpositions and in normal use of the extremity.

◀ Fig. **142** The patient shown in Figure **141** has evidence of adverse effects of cortisone treatment.

Fig. **143** Maximal possible opening of the mouth in involvement of both temporomandibular joints as a sequel of juvenile rheumatoid arthritis (same patient as in Figures **144–146**).

Fig. **144** Bony ankylosis of all joints in both hands with widespread abolition of skin creasing.

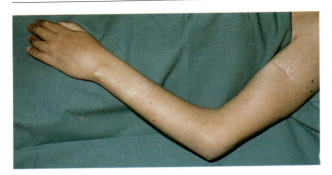

145

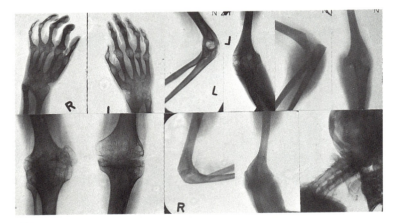

146

Fig. **145**   Bony ankylosis of the left elbow joint (also present on the right side).

Fig. **146**   Roentgenograms of several regions, some of which are in two planes, show the bony ankylosis of numerous peripheral joints, and also the cervical spine.
Center and above right: left elbow joint before and after osteotomy with interpositional arthroplasty to correct the bony ankylosis. The functional result on both sides was optimal regarding motion and lateral stability.

Other Changes

Lymph Node Swellings and Skin Lesions

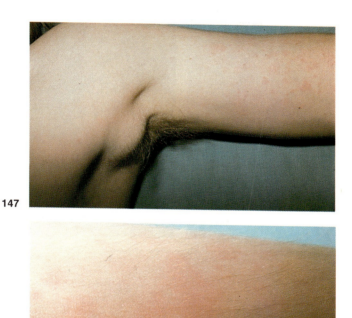

147

148

Fig. **147** Swelling of axillary lymph nodes in juvenile rheumatoid arthritis with involvement of internal organs (Still's syndrome). Mottled rheumatoid erythema multiforme on the upper arm.

Fig. **148** Blotchy confluent rheumatoid erythema multiforme on the thigh.

Treatment-Related Changes

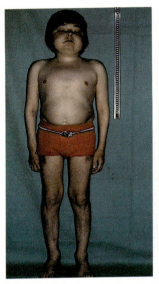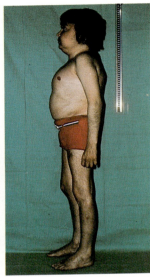

149 a + b

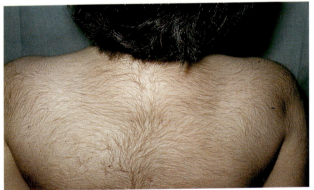

150

Figs. **149a** and **b**   20-year-old male with Still's syndrome. Stunted growth (132 cm) and other signs of hypercortisolism after receiving necessary cortisone therapy for many years.

Fig. **150**   Cortisone-induced hair growth on the back and the shoulders.

Juvenile Dematomyositis

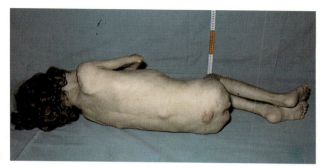

151

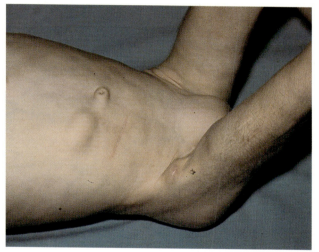

152

Fig. **151** 8-year-old girl with juvenile dermatomyositis, with flexion contractures of the large joints in the upper and lower extremities. The patient can
neither stand nor walk. There are multiple calcium deposits in the skin and the
fasciae, which are typical of this disease.

Fig. **152** Calcium deposits in the abdomen, the inguinal region, and the thigh.

Psoriatic Arthritis

Psoriatic arthritis is a chronic systemic disease with mostly concomitant psoriasis of the skin and a polyarthritis involving large, but also small, peripheral joints; it is characterized by swelling, pain, and restriction of function. Lesions of the spine (psoriatic spondylitis), amounting to ankylosis, develop in approximately 10 percent of all cases. Typical changes of the joints, but also asymmetric and rather irregular involvement (in contradistinction to rheumatoid arthritis), occasionally allow making the diagnosis when the arthritis makes its appearance before the manifestation in the skin (psoriatic arthritis without psoriasis). Subcutaneous rheumatoid nodules are absent and the rheumatoid factors is seldom demonstrable.

153

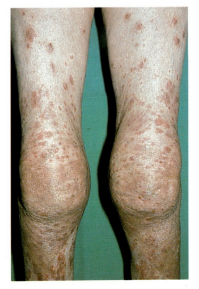

Fig. **153** Psoriasis with arthritis. Marked swelling due to synovitis, especially lateral and superior to both knee joints. Muscular atrophy is the result of immobilization because of impairment of standing and walking.

Macroscopic Features of Articular Synovitis and Tenosynovitis

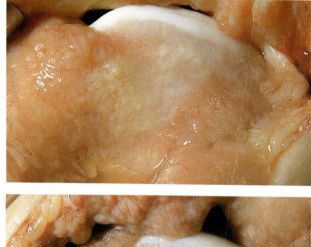

154

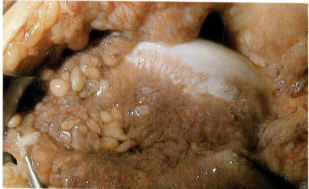

155

Fig. **154** Proliferative phase of articular synovitis of the knee joint in psioriatic arthritis. A conspicuous feature in comparison with synovitis in rheumatoid arthritis is the fact that the synovium as a whole is paler and contains more fluid. Completely intact cartilage without formation of a synovial pannus is present.

Fig. **155** Articular synovitis of the knee joint in psoriatic arthritis of longer standing. Marked formation of villi with redness of the inflamed synovial tissue, which is rarely seen in psoriatic arthritis. Distinct synovial pannus crosses the border between bone and cartilage and gives rise to destructive lesions. In the vicinity of the synovial pannus. There are isolated incipient foci of cartilage degeneration.

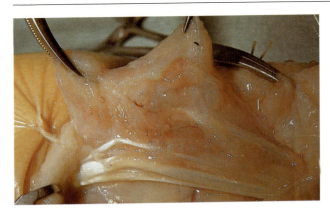

156

Fig. **156**   Tenosynovitis as a sequel of psoristic arthritis on the extensor side of the wrist under the dorsal retinaculum, which has already been opened. The inflamed synovial tissue presents a bright discoloration similar to that ir articular synovitis, and it likewise shows a conspicuous accumulation of fluid. This is the proliferative phase. However, fraying of the tendinous structure by ir filtrative growth of inflamed tensosynovial tissue is not yet demonstrable.

Fig. **157**   Deficient extensibility of the third and fourth finger of the right hand in ▶ psoriatic arthritis. This 27-year-old female stated that considerable swelling had been present on the dorsal side of the wrist over a prolonged period of time. After the inability to extend the two fingers had suddenly appeared, the swelling regressed slowly. Deficient function led to regression of the tenosynovitis. The ability to flex all fingers is not particularly restricted.

Fig. **158**   Following incision of the skin on the extensor side of the wrist, ▶ division of the dorsal retinaculum, and subsequent dissection of the individual tendon compartments, some of the tendons display a rupture. On the right side of the figure, four tendon stumps are recognizable in the tissue conglomeration. On the left side, the tendon stumps cannot be differentiated. The proximal stumps (on the left) have already been retracted a considerable distance by muscle pull. The defect between the proximal and the distal tendon stumps had been bridged by scar tissue, which probably developed from inflamed synovial tissue. Following rupture of the tendons and the subsequent functional deficiency, the inflammatory activity abates and this tissue undergoes fibrosis. The ruptured tendons belong to the following muscles: extensor digitorum communis of the third and fourth fingers, extensor carpi radialis longus and extensor carpi radialis brevis.

Synovitis-Related Changes

Tenosynovitis and its Consequences

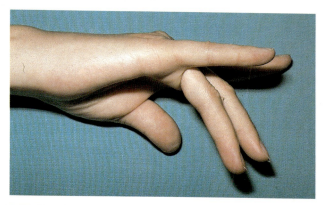

157

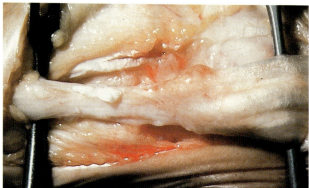

158

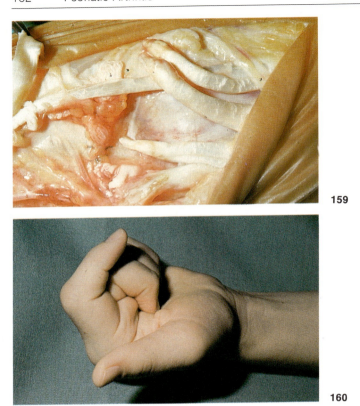

159

160

Fig. **159** The distal tendon stumps are dissected free by removing the fibrotic soft tissues and then are connected by tendon sutures to muscles that can provide energy (in the present instance, among others, the extensor indicis proprius), so that the damaged fingers, can again be extended.

Fig. **160** Tenosynovitis of the flexor tendons of the index finger with impaired flexion. Owing to adhesions of the inflamed synovial tissue to its surroundings, and also of the deep to the superficial flexor tendons at their point of penetration, complete flexion can no longer be accomplished. There remains a measurable distance between the finger end and the palm. Increase or decrease of this functional deficiency can be established by repetitive comparable measurements.

Articular Synovitis an Its Consequences

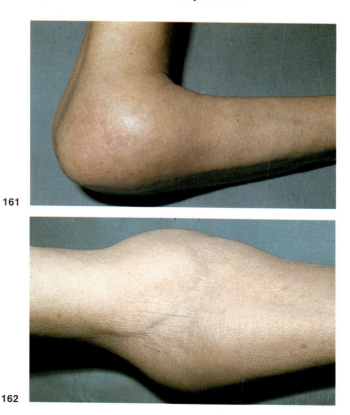

Fig. **161** Marked swelling of elbow joint during flexion, due to synovitis in psoriatic arthritis.

Fig. **162** The same elbow joint as in Fig. **161** with the forearm extended.

Typical Joint Lesions in Psoriatic Arthritis

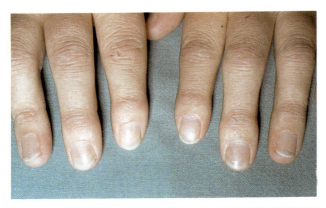

163

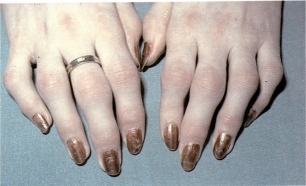

164

Fig. **163**   Multiple symmetric involvement of the distal interphalangeal joint is typical of psoriatic arthritis. This condition must not be confused with osteoarthritis of the distal interphalangeal joints, which is frequently accompanied by the formation of Heberden's nodes. In rheumatoid arthritis, the distal interphalangeal joints are relatively seldom involved.

Fig. **164**   Combined involvement of distal and proximal interphalangeal joints in psoriatic arthritis. The involvement is symmetric, whereas otherwise lesions of the small joints of hand and feet generally are asymmetric, in contradistinction to rheumatoid arthritis.

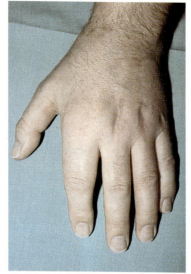

165

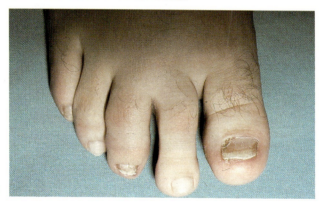

166

Fig. **165** The concomitant affection of the metacarpophalangeal and the proximal and the distal interphalangeal joints of a finger or a toe – involvement of the entire digit – is a lesion that is typical of psoriatic arthritis. With involvement of the entire digit, the soft tissues are considerably swollen, resulting in the appearance of the "sausage finger" (here the index finger).

Fig. **166** Involvement of the entire third toe ("sausage toe").

Extreme Lesions in the Region of the Hands

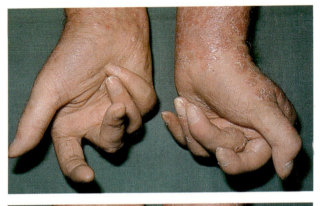

167

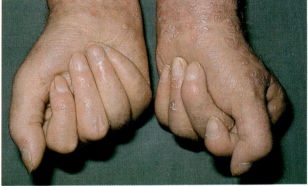

168

Fig. **167** End stage of the hands in psoriatic arthritis. The hands display considerable alterations. When the patient attempts to open his hands, extension of almost all fingers is extremely limited.

Fig. **168** In contrast, the patient can make a tight fist, but prehensile movements are considerably restricted owing to the limitations in unclenching the hands.

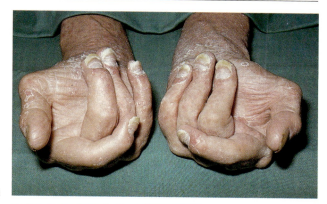

169a

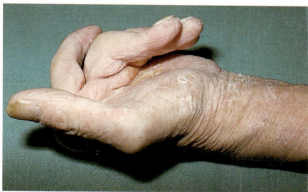

169b

Figs. **169a** and **b**   Nearly complete fixation of the three ulnar long fingers when a tight fist is made. Extreme ulnar deviation of the index fingers, both of them lying over the metacarpophalangeal joint of the third and fourth fingers. When the patient makes an attempt at unclenching his hands, the tips of the third, fourth and fifth fingers are only little raised from their supporting surface. There is marked functional impairment of both hands.

In the present case the metacarpophalangeal joints were replaced by a total prosthesis, and an arthroplasty – partly combined with arthrodesis in a position of function – was performed on some distal joints. In this way the patient was enabled after 15 years of ankylosis to make a nearly tight fist and to unclench his hands almost completely.

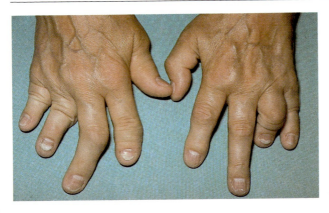

170

Fig. **170**   Advanced involvement of varying joints of several fingers in both hands. The asymmetric involvement is typical of psoriatic arthritis. The shortening of the fingers is due to mutilation of some joints.

Foot Lesions

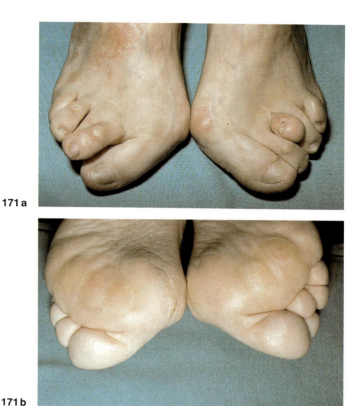

171 a

171 b

Figs. **171 a** and **b**   Fibular deviation at the metatarsophalangeal joints of all toes and development of hallux valgus can also occur in psoriatic arthritis. Marked callosities on the sole as the result of articular synovitis of all the metatarsophalangeal joints.

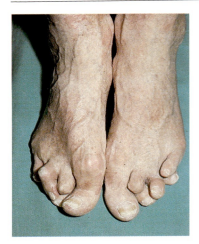

172

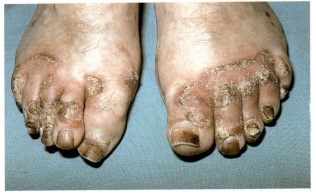

173

Fig. **172**   Asymmetric lesions of both feet with a double right-angled deformity of the great toe. Buttonhole deformity of individual small toes is seen.

Fig. **173**   Incipient buttonhole deformity of individual toes. Extensive psoriatic foci. Black discoloration of the nails is the result of potassium permanganate foot baths.

Lesions of Skin and Nails in Psoriatic Arthritis

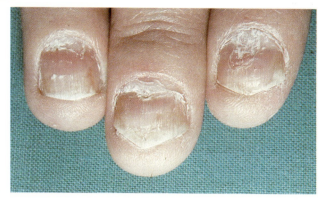

174

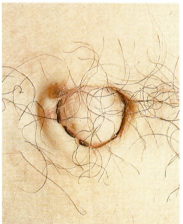

175

Fig. **174**   Even when a suspicion of psoriatic arthritis is entertained, the corresponding lesions of the skin and its appendages should be looked for in psoriatic arthritis: the fingernails present an uneven surface and part of the nail plate is friable. In addition, so-called oil stains are encountered. Discrete skin lesions are found in the locations depicted in Figures **175–177.**

Fig. **175**   Isolated skin lesions are frequently present in the umbilical region.

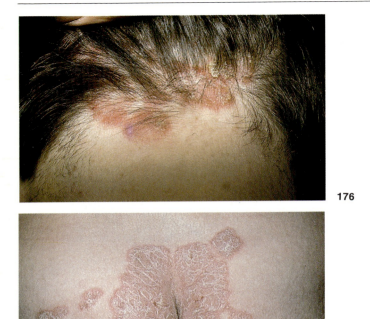

176

177

Fig. **176**   Lesions at the hairline in the back of the neck.

Fig. **177**   Involvement of the rima ani.

Ankylosing Spondylitis

Ankylosing spondylitis is a chronic inflammatory, partly destructive and partly metaplastic-productive systemic disease that affects chiefly the spine but also peripheral joints. It has a tendency to ankylosis. In more than 90 percent of all cases HLA-B27 is demonstrable.

Spinal Lesions

Clinical Changes and Their Consequences

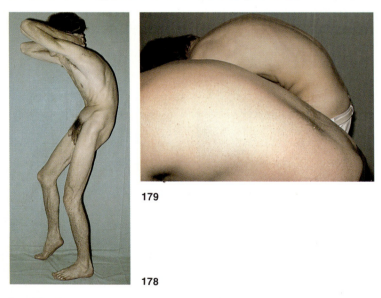

179

178

Fig. **178** Patient with ankylosing spondylitis presenting a (possibly avoidable) extreme kyphosis and a flexion contracture of the hip joints. The contracture is more marked on the right side and therefore has led to shortening of the right leg. The shortening was equalized by a reactive talipes equinus position.

Fig. **179** Difference between flexibility and extensibility of the spine in a healthy individual (behind) and in a patient with spondylitis (in front). The latter exhibits conspicuous flattening and absent extensibility of the spine.

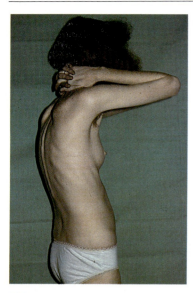

Fig. **180**   In females, the disease more often runs an abortive, and thereby more favorable, course than in males. On this account, it is frequently not recognized. Advanced lesions of the spine and the peripheral joints are much less often seen.

Figs. **181 a** and **b**   The consequence of stiffening of the spine and the thorax is the abdominal type of respiration.
a) on inspiration
b) on expiration.

180
181 a
181 b

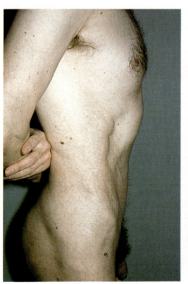

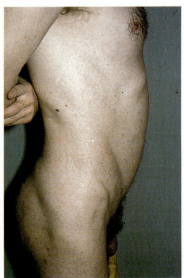

Radiologic Changes

Fig. **182** Radiologic picture of full-blown ankylosing spondylitis in the thoracic and lumbar spine with bridging syndesmophytes and ultimate development of a bamboo spine.

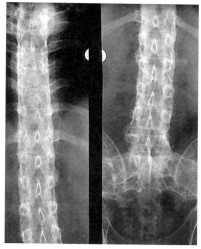

182

Fig. **183** Inflammation-dependent bilateral remodeling and bony ankylosis of the sacroiliac joints.

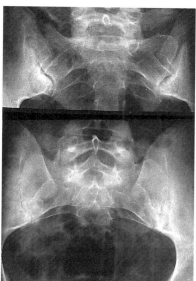

183

Lesions of the Peripheral Joints

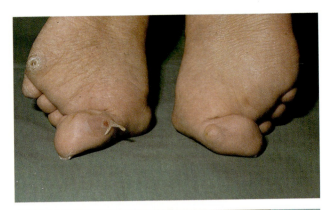

184

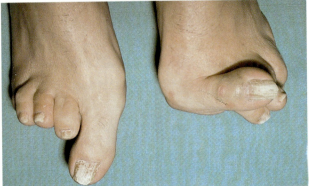

185

Fig. **184** Development of bilateral hallux valgus, fibular deviation, and dorsal dislocation of the toes II–V, multiple bursae, callosities, and ulcerations as the result of deformations and the consequent conditions of anomalous pressure in the regions of the feet, which are chiefly exposed to strain.

Fig. **185** Superduction and fibular deviation is more marked in the left hallux than in the other toes. Dorsal dislocation of all small toes with shortening of the feet.

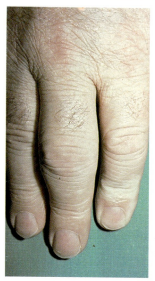

Figs. **186a** and **b** Synovitis of the third right proximal interphalangeal joint with incipient buttonhole deformity.

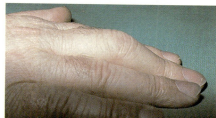

186a

186b

Fig. **187** Swan-neck deformity of several fingers of both hands.

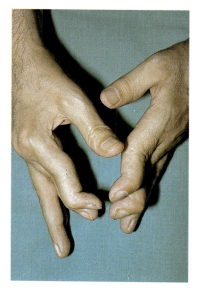

187

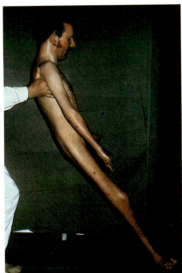

Extreme Lesions

Fig. **188**   Nearly all spinal and peripheral joints have undergone bony ankylosis. The patient can only lie down and stand.

Figs. **189a** and **b**   Advanced lesions, particularly of the cervical and the thoracic spine, in a 58-year-old female with ankylosing spondylitis.

188
189a   **189b**

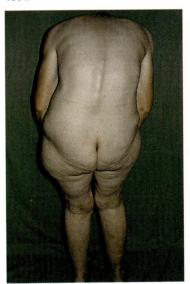

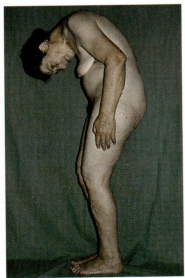

Reiter's Disease

Reiter's disease is characterized by the triad:
– arthritis,
– conjunctivitis, and
– urethritis.
There exist relationships with preceding infections. In more than one third of the cases the syndrome appears in an incomplete form, i.e., one of the manifestations (usually conjunctivitis) is lacking. Some patients show a continuous transition to classic ankylosing spondylitis, whereas in other patients involvement of the peripheral joints prevails.

Synovitis-Induced Clinical Changes

Articular Synovitis

Fig. **190**   Relatively infrequent occurrence of arthritis in the distal interphalangeal joint of the index finger with development of a sausage finger in Reiter's disease.

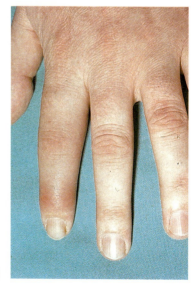

190

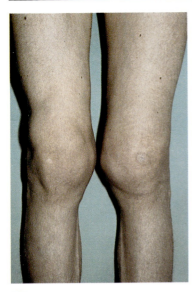

Fig. **191**   A more frequent event is synovitis in the joints of the lower extremities – here the left knee joint – with obliteration of the contours.

Fig. **192**   Reiter's disease can produce concomitant arthritis of several joints of the lower extremities, for example the right knee joint, with considerable enlargement of the upper recess.

191
192   **193**

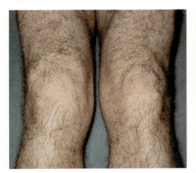

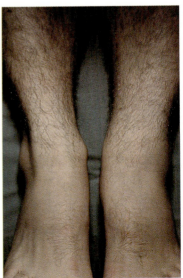

Fig. **193**   Swelling of the left tibiotalar joint in the early stage of Reiter's disease.

Tenosynovitis

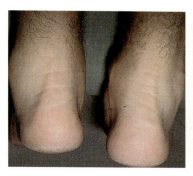

194

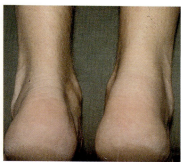

195

Fig. **194**   Swelling of the ankle joint spreading dorsally to the calcaneal grooves and the Achilles tendon.

Fig. **195**   Conspicuous inflammation of the glide tissue of the right Achilles tendon in Reiter's disease.

196

Bursitis

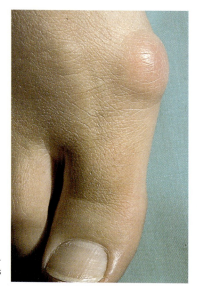

Fig. **196**   Bursitis over the metatarsophalangeal joint of the great toe as part of Reiter's syndrome.

Extrasynovial Lesions

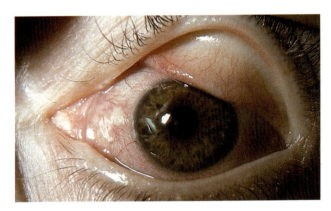

197

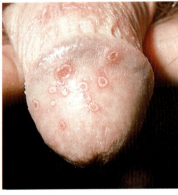

198

Fig. **197** Conjunctivitis with concomitant arthritis and urethritis in Reiter's syndrome.

Fig. **198** Circinate balanitis with slightly raised borders of the rounded foci, an involvement of the mucosa that is frequently observed in Reiter's disease.

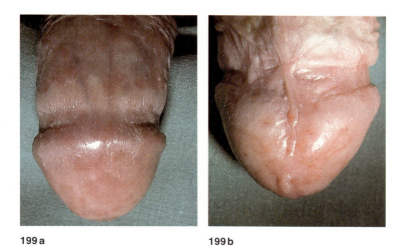

199 a   **199 b**

Figs. **199a** and **b**   Balanitis in the healing stage (same patient as in Figs. **192** and **193**).

Other "Rheumatic" Lesions and Affections in the Region of the Hand

Osteoarthritis

Interphalangeal Joints

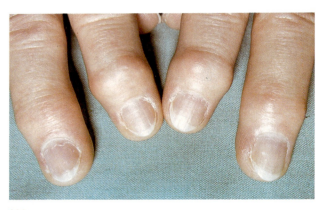

200

201   **202**

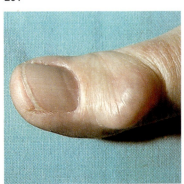

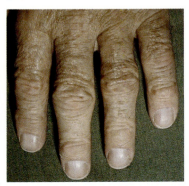

Multiple Osteoarthritis of the Hand

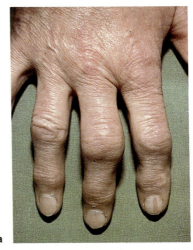

Figs. **203a** and **b**   Multiple osteoarthritis of the hand. Combination of Bouchard's and Heberden's osteoarthritis.   **203a**

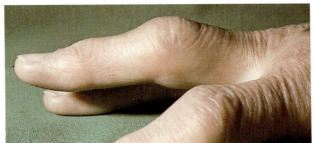

203b

Fig. **200**   Heberden's nodes on the dorsal aspects of the distal interphalangeal joints with osteoarthritis of these joints. Like all osteoarthritis lesions of the hand, Heberden's nodes appear predominantly in women at the time of menopause. The nodes are often associated with radiologically demonstrable osteoarthritis of the distal interphalangeal joints.

Fig. **201**   In so-called Heberden's osteoarthritis – here of the interphalangeal joint of the hallux – mucous cysts are occasionally encountered (dorsal cysts, parasynovial cysts), which contain mucin or hyaluronic acid.

Fig. **202**   Incipient Bouchard's osteoarthritis (degenerative lesions of the proximal interphalangeal joints). It is rather uncommon for this disorder to occur in an isolated form; it is usually associated with Heberden's osteoarthritis.

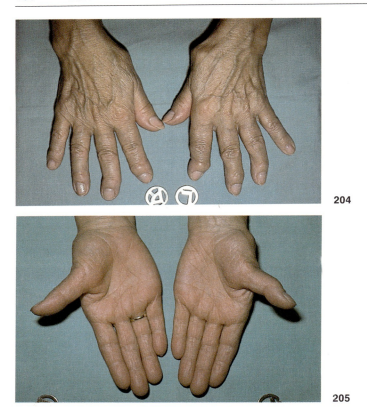

204

205

Fig. **204**   Deficient extension and lateral deviation of some of the distal inter-phalangeal joints as a sequel of Heberden's osteoarthritis. Conspicuous promi-nence of the base of the first metacarpal in both hands with concomitant adduction contracture — due to degenerative lesions and insufficiency of ligaments of the first carpometacarpal joint — as a manifestation of osteoarthritis of the saddle joint of the thumb.

Fig. **205**   Osteoarthritis of the saddle joint of the thumb leads to adduction contracture of the first metacarpal. To equalize this limitation of function, the thumb develops a reactive hyperextensibility at its metacarpophalangeal joint. Grip strength and opposition of the thumb are restored by this ability for equalization.

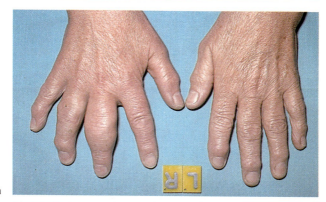

206 a

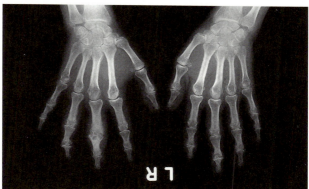

206 b

Figs. **206 a** and **b** Destructive multiple lesions of osteoarthritis of the third proximal interphalangeal joint of the right hand and with extreme thickening of the bones and soft tissue in the entire surroundings. Otherwise largely inconspicuous Heberden's and Bouchard's osteoarthritis of the distal and proximal interphalangeal joints and the saddle joint of the thumb. Besides the purely degenerative lesions of these joints, which are recognizable in the roentgenogram, destruction with cystic erosions is visible in the third right proximal interphalangeal joint.

Lesions of the Soft Tissues

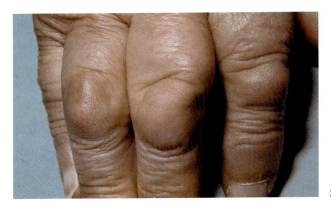

207

Fig. **207**   Knuckle pads, which often present a slight reddish or even darker discoloration, are harmless asymptomatic thickenings over the dorsal aspects of the knuckles, usually the proximal interphalangeal joints. A Dupuytren's contracture is frequently encountered concomitantly.

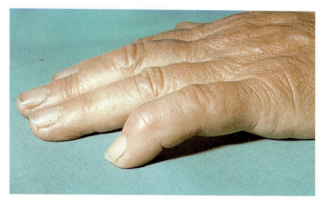

208

Fig. **208**   Slightly reddened swelling of the dorsal aspect of the fifth inter-phalangeal joint. The distal phalanx, which is in a position of flexion, cannot be extended as the consequence of subcutaneous rupture of the extensor tendon at its insertion in the base of the distal phalanx, due to a degenerative process. This injury is triggered, but not caused, by a relatively excessive strain produced by sudden pressure on the tip of the completely extended finger. The accident occurs frequently in elderly females while planting flowers, piling or sorting linen, or tucking sheets under a mattress.

Other Connective Tissue Disorders

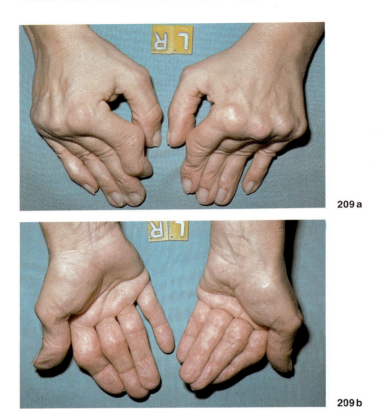

209a

209b

Figs. **209a** and **b**   Hyperflexibility of the joints, in the present case limited chiefly to the hands, occurring in the setting of an Ehlers-Danlos syndrome. The disorder has led to dislocation of the metacarpophalangeal joints and to the development of a swan-neck deformity. The Ehlers-Danlos syndrome is a generalized fibrous dysplasia that, among other features, is characterized by hyperelasticity of the skin and hypermobility of the joints.

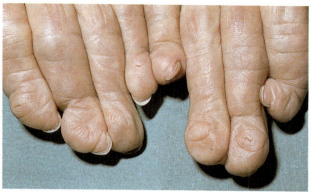

210

Fig. **210**   Cutis hyperelastica. In the Ehlers-Danlos syndrome the skin can be pulled from the underlying structures in large folds. The hyperelasticity of the skin, which is due to a collagen defect that involves the arrangement of the fibrils into bundles, decreases its inherent contractility to such a degree that otherwise trivial post-traumatic and post-operative hemorrhages lead to large hematomas. (This happened in some patients on whom we have operated.) The skin itself is soft and fragile and becomes readily torn.

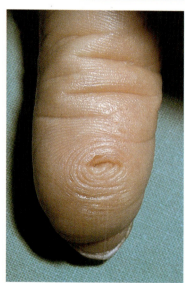

211

Fig. **211**   Prominent epidermal ridges in the fingertips.

Neurovascular Lesions

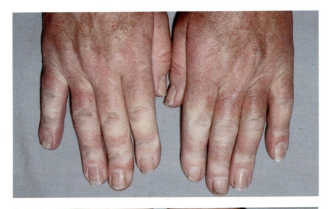

212a

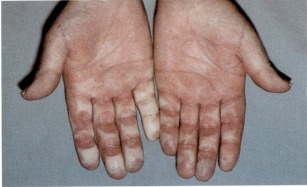

212b

Figs. **212a** and **b** Raynaud's disease in a 60-year-old female. Alternating hyperemic and blanched areas provoked by emersion in cold water and subsequently making a fist. The symptoms also occur in cold water. There is no basis for the assumption of an underlying disease.

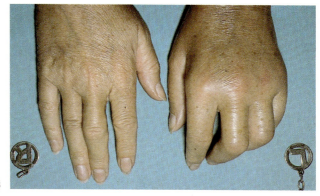

213

Fig. **213** A 54-year-old female with Sudeck's dystrophy following operation for Dupuytren's contracture and subsequent immobilization. The condition is characterized by extreme edema of soft tissues, cold glossy skin, pain, and considerable impairment of function. Sudeck's dystrophy frequently occurs postoperatively after trauma, and it mostly occurs in mentally unstable patients without authoritative guidance. The disorder is classified among the algodystrophies or reflex dystrophies.

Peripheral Nerve Compression Syndromes

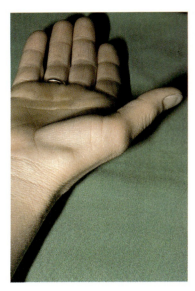

Fig. **214**   60-year-old female with marked atrophy of the thenar eminence of the right hand, as well as nocturnal paresthesias and pain radiating distally and proximally. In the early morning, impairment of prehensile movements and apposition of the thumb. The patient has difficulty in holding a toothbrush, a coffee cup, or the paper: carpal tunnel syndrome.

214

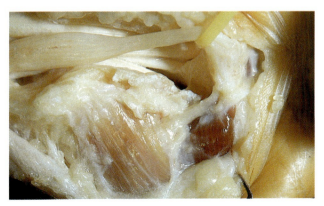

215

Collagen Diseases in the Narrow Sense

These diseases include a number of connective tissue disorders with involvement of joints and leading to fibrinoid degeneration and necrosis of collagenous fibrils, which can be demonstrated histologically. Many of these collagen diseases carry a poor prognosis.

◀ Fig. **215** Operative finding in the carpal tunnel syndrome, one of the peripheral nerve compression syndromes. All of them are due to purely mechanical compression of a peripheral nerve. The median nerve has been looped; the effect of its being compressed under the resected transverse carpal ligament is distinctly visible. The rests of the ligament can be recognized between the compressed nerve and the atrophic muscles of the thenar which are innervated by the median nerve and which display a bright appearance resembling fish flesh. Proximally to the ligament, the nerve is greatly distended. At the level of the yellow loop, the motor twig for the thenar branches in an arc from the median nerve to the left and downward to disappear in the atrophic musculature.

Scleroderma
Lesions of the Hands

Incipient Lesions of the Hands

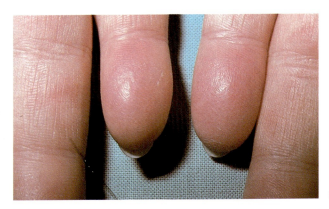

216

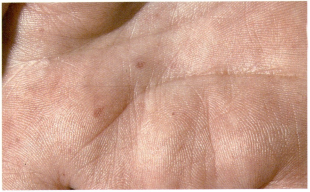

217

Fig. **216**   Erythema in the region of individual fingertips as an early sign of scleroderma in a 43-year-old female. Scleroderma is a connective tissue disease due to disordered collagen metabolism of the vessels and the interstitium. It involves the skin, the mucosa, the joints, and subsequently also the internal organs.

Fig. **217**   60-year-old female with teleangiectasias in the palm in Raynaud's disease. Suspicion as to the existence of scleroderma or the CRST syndrome (**C**alcinosis, **R**aynaud's phenomenon, **S**clerodactyly, **T**eleangiectasias). The CRST syndrome is also classified among the collagen diseases.

Advanced Lesions of the Hands

Clinical Changes

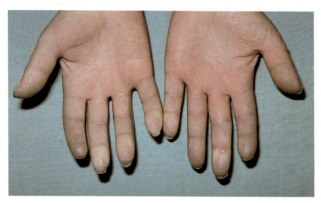

218

Fig. **218**   A 67-year-old female has had sensory disturbances in the hands, the feet, and the face for about 17 years. Scleroderma has given rise to induration of the skin and lesions in the fingertips that resemble damage done by mice. Cold provokes a violaceous or even white discoloration, especially of the acral parts.

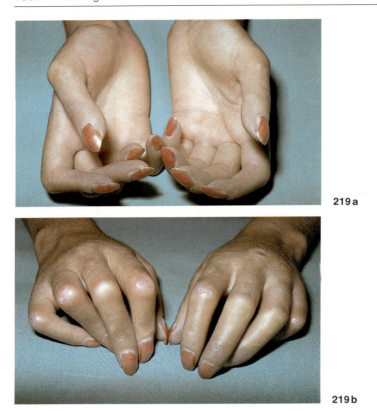

219a

219b

Figs. **219a** and **b**   38-year-old female patient with advanced sclerodactyly. The skin is considerably indurated and is barely or not at all movable against the underlying tissues. Scars from ulcerations are visible on the dorsal aspects of individual finger joints. Primarily, extension, but also flexion of the fingers at the individual joints, is considerably restricted. The residual movements are rigid. The soft tissues taper distally with flattening of the fingertips, resulting in the so-called Madonna-like hand. The restricted mobility of the fingers leads to the development of a claw hand.

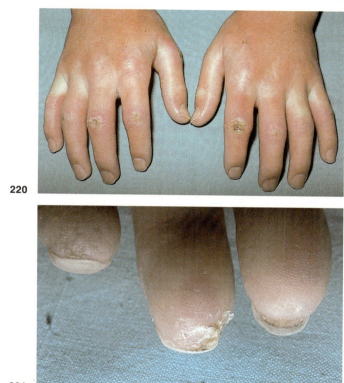

220

221

Fig. **220** Raynaud's phenomenon and marked deep ulcerations over the dorsal aspects of the proximal interphalangeal joints and abolition of skin creasing in scleroderma.

Fig. **221** So-called rat bite scars following necrosis of the fingertips and bulging of the nails. These lesions can lead to deformation resembling a bird's claw.

Radiologic Changes

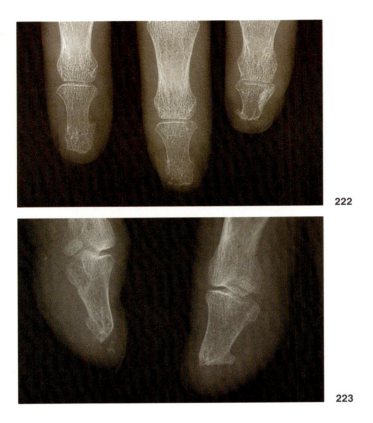

222

223

Fig. **222** Atrophy of the soft tissues of the fingertips with incipient or advanced osteolysis of the nail bed.

Fig. **223** Acral osteolysis of the distal phalanges of both thumbs with calcifications in the region of the fingertips and the distal phalanges in scleroderma.

Oral Lesions

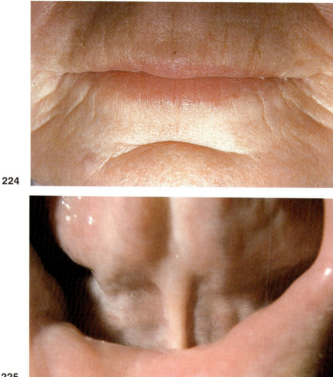

224

225

Fig. **224** Radiate creasing of the mouth with a feeling of tension. The increasing pursestring lesion interferes with opening of the mouth and eventually leads to microstoma.

Fig. **225** Strongly thickened and shortened tendinous frenum of the tongue.

Circumscribed Scleroderma

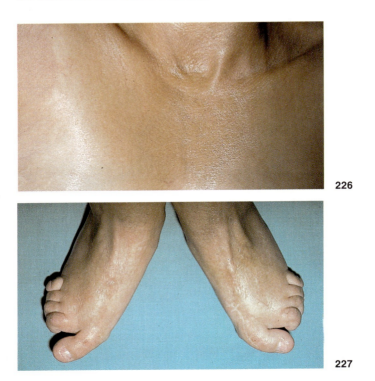

226

227

Fig. **226**   Circumscribed scleroderma (morphea) with lesions in the regions of the chest and the neck in a 35-year-old female. Morphea is not associated with involvement of internal organs and therefore carries a more favorable prognosis than progressive (systemic) scleroderma.

Fig. **227**   Lesions of the skin and the toes in the patient depicted in Figure **226**. Fibular deviation of all toes, in the left foot following unsuccessful operation on the great toe, and development of claw toes. Resection of the metatarsal heads of all toes and resection of the heads of the proximal phalanges of the eight small toes plus a temporary arthrodesis with use of crossed wires – operations that are also performed in rheumatoid arthritis – produced a considerable and painless improvement of gait, also by increasing the capability of heel-toe walking. Since then, the patient can wear fashionable ready-made shoes and boots. Orthopedic shoes are no longer required.

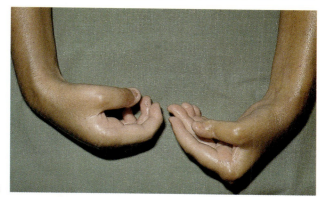

228 a

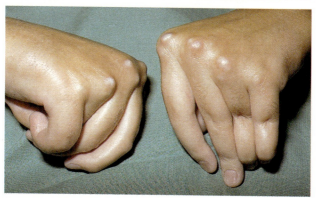

228 b

Fig. **228 a** and **b**   Deformity of the hands similar to the changes in rheumatoid arthritis. The patient is the same as in Figure **226**. Fixed flexed position of both wrist joints, double right-angled deformity of the left thumb, ulnar deviation, and dislocation of the long fingers at the metacarpophalangeal joints, and stiffening or ankylosis of several interphalangeal joints with development of a swan-neck deformity in some of them are present.

Arthrodesis of the wrists and individual interphalangeal joints in the so-called position of function, as well as total arthroplasty of the metacarpophalangeal joints after Swanson, produced an improvement of function. Operation on the extremities are not often indicated in scleroderma. They should be reserved for the specialist experienced in orthopedic surgery of the arthritic patient.

Polymyositis and Dermatomyositis

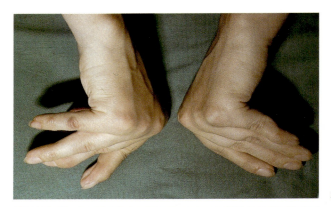

229 a

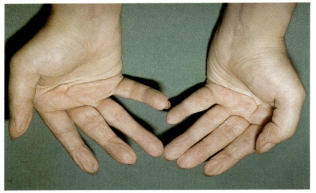

229 b

Figs. **229 a** and **b**　22-year-old female with dermatomyositis, an autoimmune collagen disease, and Ehlers-Danlos syndrome. Subluxation and ulnar deviation of the long fingers at the metacarpophalangeal joints results in considerable impairment of extension. Several fingers present a swan-neck deformity that, however, can be functionally equalized to a great extent. Polymyositis and dermatomyositis are accompanied by involvement of joints without destruction, but particularly by changes in the musculature progressing to atrophy, and by skin lesions.

Polymyalgia Rheumatica

This disorder probably develops on the basis of generalized immunologic vascular damage. It can often be diagnosed by the concomitant occurrence of temporal arteritis (giant cell arteritis) associated with extreme elevation of the erythrocyte sedimentation rate and pains in the shoulder girdle.

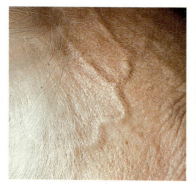 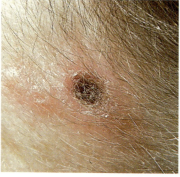

230 **231**

Fig. **230** Strongly thickened, tortuous temporal artery showing little pulsation. At the same time, there is localized pain and pain in the muscles of the shoulder girdle. Extreme elevation of the erythrocyte sedimentation rate and its decrease as well as the abatement of pain that followed high-dose cortisone therapy confirmed the diagnosis of polymyalgia rheumatica.

Fig. **321** Dry necrosis with surrounding erythema as the result of deficient perfusion in the region supplied by the temporal artery.

Rheumatic Diseases of Metabolism

Gout

Gout is a metabolic disease characterized by acute attacks but some-times also by a steady course, which affects males with much greater frequency than females. Initially, the disease has a marked preference for the metatarsophalangeal joint of the great toes. Uric acid crystals are deposited in the region of the joint, especially the synovial tissue. Tophi develop and destruction of joints occurs in untreated patients. Hyperuricemia is present in most cases.

Foot Lesions

Podagra

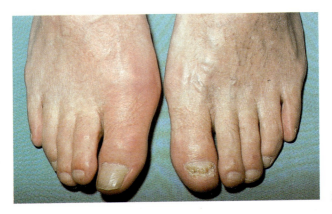

232

Fig. **232** First gouty attack in a 59-year-old male with sudden appearance of extreme pain in the metatarsophalangeal joint of the right great toe, accompanied by redness and swelling. Standing and walking were nearly impossible. Elevation of the foot and application of cold had some alleviating effect. During the attack, the serum value of uric acid was 8.31 mg per cent or 494 µmol/liter.

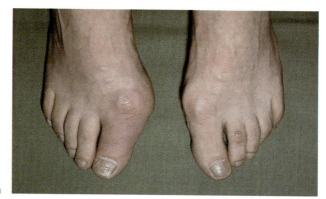

233a

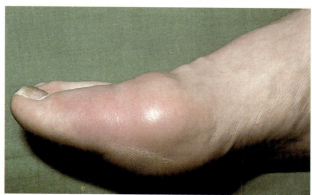

233b

Fig. **233** 51-year-old male with repeated gouty attacks in the region of the right great toe. Osteoarthritis of the metatarsophalangeal joint has already developed. A small gouty tophus is present on the dorsal aspect of the second left proximal interphalangeal joint.

Other Foot Lesions

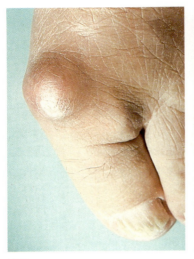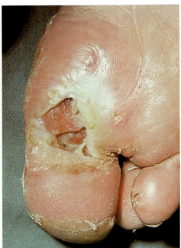

234   **235**

Fig. **234** Bursitis over the first metatarsophalangeal joint in chronic gout.

Fig. **235** Deep ulcer as the sequel of a superinfected, spontaneously perforating tophus on the plantar aspect of the metatarsophalangeal joint of the great toe.

Figs. **236a** and **b** A 52-year-old man with gout was referred for amputation because of extreme bulbous enlargement, heat, and intense redness of his third toe. Pus (containing Staphylococcus aureus) and whitish pulpous tophaceous masses were discharged through a number of spontaneous perforations (one of them on the lateral side of the nail).
Following incision with antibiotic coverage, the tophus and the necrotic tissue were removed. This was followed by primary closure with prolonged suction drainage. The toe was salvaged by this procedure.

Fig. **237** Confluent gouty tophi above and in front of the left external malleolus.

Fig. **238** Multiple tophi in the regions of the heels and the Achilles tendons.

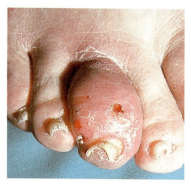

236 a

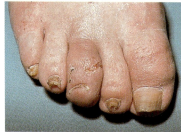

236 b

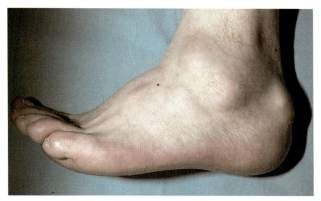

237

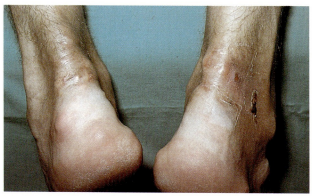

238

Lesions of the Hand

Cheiragra

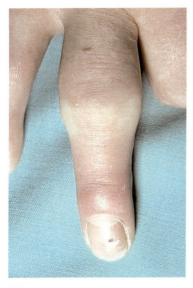

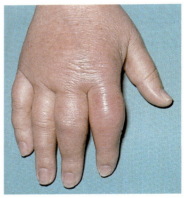

239   **240**

Fig. **239**   Acute attack of gouty arthritis of the third distal interphalangeal joint with involvement of the third proximal interphalangeal joint of some duration in a 31-year-old male.

Fig. **240**   62-year-old female with acute gouty arthritis of the second proximal interphalangeal joint and elevated uric acid values. Besides this, the patient has rheumatoid arthritis; the latter has occasioned, among other lesions, a synovitis of the third proximal interphalangeal joint with incipient buttonhole deformity. The difference between the two types of arthritis is obvious: the index finger presents manifestations of an acute inflammation with strong spontaneous pain, increased heat, bulbous distention of the entire surroundings of the joint, and thin glossy skin with nearly complete abolition of creasing. The third proximal interphalangeal joint shows a circumscribed swelling that is due to herniation of synovial tissue that has perforated the dorsal aponeurosis. Continuous pain, particularly on motion, although of much less intensity than that in the second proximal interphalangeal joint. Concomitant affliction with gout and rheumatoid arthritis is rare.

Other Lesions in the Region of the Hand

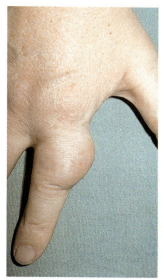

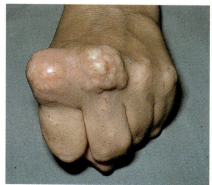

Fig. **241** Development of a tophus over the metacarpophalangeal joint of the second right finger. No signs of acute inflammation, but there is irritation of branches of the radial nerve for the fingers.

Fig. **242** Multiple tophi on the dorsal aspects of the hands, as well as the feet.

Fig. **243** Loculation is visible when the patient clenches his left fist. In the absence of a spontaneous tendency to regression. Extirpation of the tophus is indicated because of threatened perforation.

Miniature Tophi

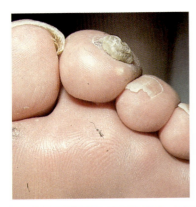

244

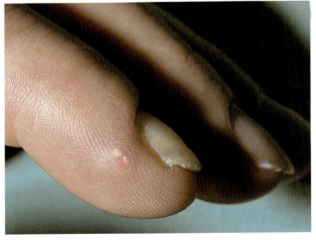

245

Fig. **244**   Miniature tophus on the tip of the second toe.

Fig. **245**   Small tophus on the radial side of the tip of the index finger; intermittent spontaneous perforation.

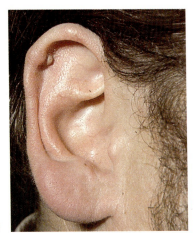

246

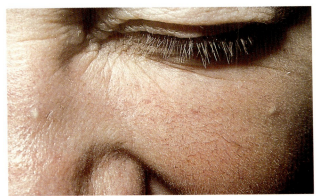

247

Fig. **246**   Tophus of typical location on the right auricle.

Fig. **247**   In gout, intracutaneous miniature tophi are occasionally encountered in the face (in the nose and the cheeks).

Lesions of Bursae

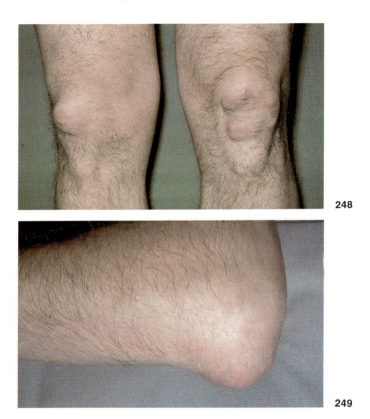

248

249

Fig. **248**   Multiple occurrence of, partly loculated, bursitis and gouty tophi in the region of both knee joints.

Fig. **249**   Gouty olecranon bursitis.

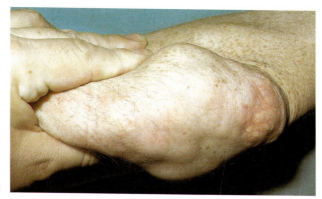

250

Fig. **250** Extensive olecranon bursitis with large amounts of uric acid, much of it embedded in the wall. The bursa is loculated; a perforation is present in its cranial portion. The uric acid deposits there can be recognized through the skin.

Chondrocalcinosis

Chondrocalcinosis is a polyarticular affection characterized by an episodic and chronic course. It is nearly always accompanied by degenerative changes in the diseased joints, in the cartilage of which calcium pyrophosphate crystals are deposited.

Macroscopic Lesions of Joints

251

252

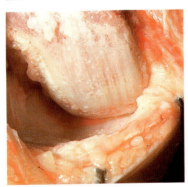
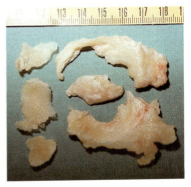

Fig. **251** Chondrocalcinosis (calcium gout, pseudogout) with calcium pyrophosphate embedded in the cartilage, which has degenerative changes. Secondary osteoarthritis with signs of abrasion are present. Chondrocalcinosis is a polyarticular affection characterized by an episodic and chronic course. It is

Radiologic Changes

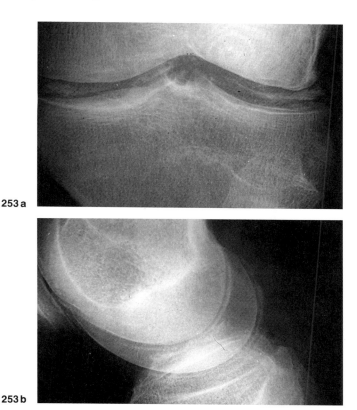

253a

253b

nearly always accompanied by degenerative changes in the diseased joints in the cartilage of which calcium pyrophosphate crystals are deposited.

◀ Fig. **252** Embeddings of calcium pyrophosphate in the articular cartilage and the menisci.

Figs. **253a** and **b** The embedding of calcium pyrophosphate in the hyaline articular cartilage is recognizable by a delicate linear or punctate shadow (Dihlmann) The shadow runs, as a characteristic feature, parallel to the bony surface.

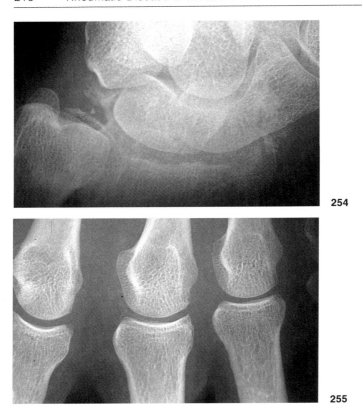

254

255

Fig. **254** The region of the wrist also reveals a linear deposit of calcium salts, which runs parallel to the border of the bone. In addition, cloudy deposits are found in fibrocartilage (e.g., the disks and the menisci), in the present case in the ulnar and the radial regions of the joint.

Fig. **255** Delicate contours in the regions of the finger joints are encountered much less frequently.

Ochronosis

Ochronosis is a metabolic disease that is accompanied by alkaptonuria. A brown-black derivative of homogentisic acid is deposited in bradytrophic mesenchymal tissues (e.g., cartilage and joint capsule) or increased amounts of it are excreted in the urine.

Macroscopic Lesions of Joints

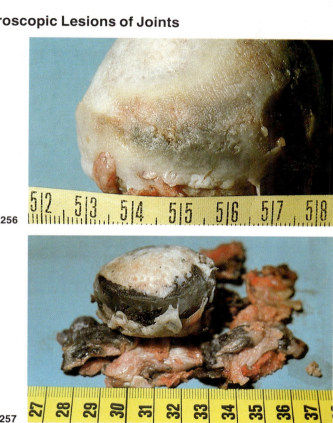

Fig. **256**   Ochronotic discoloration of the articular cartilage.

Fig. **257**   Not only the parts of the femoral head which are still covered with cartilage but also the synovial and the fibrous capsule of the hip joint are – at least partly – affected by the dark discoloration. Noncartilaginous parts of the femoral head, its "bald part" reveal no deposit of ochronotic pigment.

Other Changes

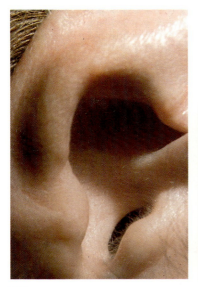

258

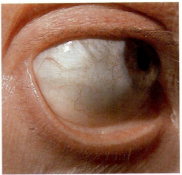

259

Fig. **258** Brownish shimmer in the region of the auricle is a manifestation of pigment deposition.

Fig. **259** Brownish discoloration from ochronosis. Pigment is also encountered in the visible parts of the sclera.

Hemochromatosis

Hemochromatosis is a disorder of iron metabolism with an accumulation of ferrous pigment in parenchymatous and mesenchymatous tissues.

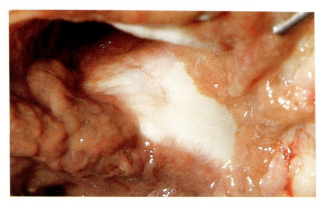

260

Fig. **260** Chronic synovitis of the knee joint with an acute, painful episode of prolonged duration in hemochromatosis. Intense brown discoloration of the inflamed synovial tissue.

Fig. **261** Besides hepatomegaly, diabetes mellitus, elevated serum levels of iron and ferritin, it is initially the pigmentation of the skin (bronze diabetes) that suggests the correct diagnosis.

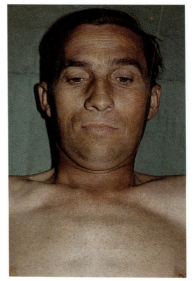

261

References

Albrecht, H. J.: Rheumatologie für die Praxis. Karger, Basel 1975

Bach, G. L., F. Schilling: Kennbilder der wichtigsten rheumatischen Erkrankungen. Eular, Basel 1977

Boyle, A. C.: A Colour Atlas of Rheumatology, 2nd ed. Wolfe, London 1980

Dihlmann, W.: Gelenke, Wirbelverbindungen. Klinische Radiologie, 2nd ed. Thieme, Stuttgart 1982

Dihlmann, W.: Therapie der entzündlich-rheumatischen Krankheiten. Mediamed, Ravensburg 1983

Dihlmann, W., H. Mathies: Das rheumatische Gelenk. Sharp & Dohme, München 1976

Faßbender, H. G.: Pathologie rheumatischer Erkrankungen. Springer, Berlin 1972

Gschwend, N.: Die operative Behandlung der progressiv chronischen Polyarthritis, 2nd ed. Thieme, Stuttgart 1977

Hornstein, O. P.: Veränderungen der Haut und der Mundschleimhaut bei rheumatischen Erkrankungen. Eular, Basel 1980

Kaiser, H.: Rheuma – ein Symptom. Editiones Roche, Basel 1982

Kölle, G.: Die juvenile rheumatoide Arthritis und das Still-Syndrom. Rheumaforum 4. Braun, Karlsruhe 1975

Korting, G. W., H. Holzmann: Die Sklerodermie und ihr nahestehende Bindegewebsprobleme. Thieme, Stuttgart 1967

Mathies, H.: Handbuch der inneren Medizin, vol. VI A–C. Springer, Berlin 1983/1984

Mathies, H., P. Otte, J. Villioumey, A. St. Dixon: Klassifikation der Erkrankungen des Bewegungsapparates. Eular, Basel 1978

Miehlke, K., D. Wessinghage: Entzündlicher Rheumatismus. Die Rheumafibel 1, 3rd ed. Springer, Berlin 1976

Mohr, W.: Gelenkkrankheiten. Thieme, Stuttgart 1984

Müller, W., F. Schilling: Differentialdiagnose rheumatischer Erkrankungen, 2nd ed. Aesopus, Basel 1982

Störig, E.: Rheuma-Orthopädie. Perimed, Erlangen 1982

Wessinghage, D.: Rheuma – Welche Diagnose stellen Sie? 2nd ed., Ciba-Geigy, Wehr-Basel 1980

Wessinghage, D.: Chronisch-entzündliche Gelenkerkrankungen. MMW Medizin, München 1980

Wessinghage, D.: Rheumatologie – Diasammlung mit Begleittext. Rocom, Basel 1981

Wessinghage, D., K. Miehlke: Die chronische Polyarthritis. Veränderungen, operative und konservative Behandlung. Ergebn. inn. Med. Kinderheilk. 26 (1974)

List of Names in the Historical Section

Acknowledgement of the Sources of Illustrations in the Historical Section of this Book

Figures 35, 37, 41 and 51 in the historical section were taken from the book

Garrison, F. H.:   An Introduction to the History of Medicine, W. B. Saunders Comp., Philadelphia and London, 1913.

Figure 44 was taken from the book

Valentin, B.:   Geschichte der Orthopädie, Thieme Verlag, Stuttgart

The originals of all other historical illustrations reproduced here are from the author's own archive of the history of medicine.

Index